The
Yoga of Eating

The
Yoga of Eating

Transcending Diets and Dogma
to Nourish the Natural Self

Charles Eisenstein

NewTrends Publishing, Inc.
Washington, DC

The Yoga of Eating
Transcending Diets and Dogma
to Nourish the Natural Self

Charles Eisenstein
Cover Design by Patsy Kuo Eisenstein

NewTrends Publishing, Inc.
Washington, DC   20007

www.NewTrendsPublishing.com   newtrends@kconline.com
US and Canadian Orders (877) 707-1776
International Orders (574) 268-2601

Available to the trade through
Biblio Distribution (a division of NBN) (800) 462-6420

First Printing: 10,000

ISBN   0-9670897-2-7

PRINTED IN THE UNITED STATES OF AMERICA

I must have been incredibly simple or drunk or insane
To sneak into my own house and steal money,
To climb over the fence and take my own vegetables.
But no more. I've gotten free of that ignorant fist
That was pinching and twisting my secret self.

— Jelaluddin Rumi

Yüeh: "to please" or "to delight in." The leftmost three strokes comprise the symbol for heart, while the symbol on the right means to redeem, whether cashing a check or fulfilling a promise. Together they mean to redeem what's in the heart, to appropriately match what's outside with what's inside, and thereby to take delight in the world.

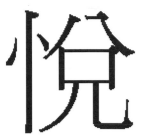

Contents

Introduction

If you are like most people, at some point in your life you will decide to improve your diet. Inspired perhaps by a health crisis or a spiritual awakening or a new relationship, you decide to eat in a healthier or more ethical way.

Unfortunately, sooner or later you are bound to discover that "improving your diet" is not as straightforward as you imagined. Buy any book on diet or nutrition and you'll find plenty of persuasive advice on what we should and should not eat. Pick up another book and you'll find equally persuasive advice in direct opposition to the first. What to do?

One book might tout the wonders of soy; another will warn us of its dangers. One book might advocate a diet consisting primarily of raw foods, rich in enzyme vitality; another advises to limit intake of raw foods, so as not to dampen the digestive fire. One book will champion honey as a super-food; another says honey is just as harmful as any other sugar. Most mainstream books on nutrition advise us limit intake of fat, particularly saturated fat; an increasingly prominent minority contends that actually, traditional animal fats are good for you. Some authorities say that supplements are absolutely essential for good health; others say they just give you "expensive urine." One philosophy might advocate a diet based on your blood type; another, based on your ayurvedic type; another, on your Chinese medicine element. Some ethical systems are based on vegetarianism, others on localism, others on specific social or environmental issues.

The examples are endless. The hapless health-food explorer faces a bewildering thicket of contradictory advice, all coming from authoritative sources. Is there one diet among them that represents the True Gospel of health—choose rightly and you are saved, choose wrongly and you'll go to health Hell? If so, how do we distinguish it from among the hundreds of other diets on offer? Or maybe they are all correct, somehow, despite their blatant contradictions. Or maybe none of them are right.

Faced with this dilemma after a decade of dietary exploration and self-experimentation, I decided to try something different. Instead of trusting any outside authority, I would trust my own body—no matter what it led me to. This decision opened up whole realms of realization and discovery: about the untapped potential of the body and its senses, about the relationship between our manner of eating and manner of being, and about the spiritual aspects of our corporeal selves. Most importantly, my practice, which I call the Yoga of Eating, freed me to enjoy, for the first time in memory, the uninhibited pleasure of food accompanied by a growing wellness and physical vitality.

I use the word "yoga" in a very general sense, to mean a practice that brings one into greater wholeness or unity. The Yoga of Eating I describe is quite distinct from "yogic diets" advocated in popular books on Hatha Yoga. I will not tell you what to eat and not to eat.

This book, then, is not a diet book, nor is it a book on nutrition. Such books have their value, of course, but they must not be taken on anyone's authority—not even if this authority represents the full weight of scientific opinion. The purpose of this book is to introduce the reader to a higher authority: your own body. But why trust your body when it seems so often to lead you astray? How can we discern what our bodies are telling us? With these questions in mind, let us now explore the philosophy and practice of the Yoga of Eating.

Chapter 1

The Fallacy of Willpower

Those who restrain desire, do so because theirs is weak enough to be restrained; and the restrainer or Reason usurps its place & governs the unwilling.
— William Blake

See how many envelopes you can lick in an hour, and in the next hour, try to beat that record!
— Principal Skinner, The Simpsons

Many people despair at the prospect of improving their eating habits, because they think they just don't have enough willpower.

Not enough willpower. How else to explain destructive dietary habits even in full knowledge of the consequences? How else to explain pigging out all day after a week of disciplined eating? How else to explain snacking on donuts after having made an earnest, well-motivated pledge to give up donuts? It appears that willpower has failed, allowing a momentary compulsion to betray us.

Our society's appeal to willpower goes far beyond diet, of course. Often we seem to think that without willpower, we'd lounge around doing nothing all day, except to fulfill our nearest needs and pleasures. "What would you do tomorrow," I ask people, "if all of a sudden you lost all your willpower?" Most people imagine sleeping in, missing work, eating a big

3

breakfast, and after that, a vague never-ending spiral of indulgence, indolence, and apathy.

Reliance on willpower reveals a profound distrust of one's self. We seem to think that what we really want to do must be bad, indulgent; therefore we must exercise willpower to enforce better behavior. Life becomes a constant regimen of "shoulds" and "shouldn'ts." But maybe this distrust is misplaced. Let's think about it more carefully: What if you really did lose your willpower tomorrow? Yes, maybe you would sleep in—but is that laziness, or a genuine need for rest? Maybe you would miss work—but couldn't that mean your work is not your soul's true work, and no longer do you force yourself to do it? You might stay in bed until ten, even until twelve, but eventually the bed would become uncomfortable. You might sit around doing nothing for a while, eating chocolate bon-bons and watching television, but eventually you'd become restless. Without work and chores to do, escapism loses its appeal. Maybe you'd feel free to catch up on neglected areas of your life. Maybe you would spend all day with your child, or a friend, or in nature. Maybe you would take up a creative project you'd never had time and energy to do. Maybe this creative project would turn into a new career, a job that you are excited to wake up to. Maybe, just maybe, life without willpower would be more creative, more abundant, more productive, and more dynamic than the life of shoulds and shouldn'ts.

The proper function of willpower and self-discipline is to extend wisdom and insight into times of imperfect clarity; to remember and apply the messages of one's inner voice. For example, if you are engaged in joyful work, when distractions come you may need to remind yourself of what you really want to be doing. Or maybe you need to remind yourself of the happiness of quiet time with family when the titillations of consumer culture beckon. In marriage, if you can remember the lightness and ease of not maintaining lies and secrets, then sexual infidelity loses its allure. And in eating, as we will see, discipline comes naturally when we integrate into present awareness the full experience of food. True discipline is really just self-remembering; no forcing or fighting is necessary.

4

When used in this way—to remember oneself, to come back into alignment—willpower is natural and energizing, whereas when we are fighting ourselves, it is an ordeal. Often we use "self-discipline" to tell our inner voice to shut up, preferring to trust in the rational mind and its received beliefs. This is unfortunate: What if our inner appetites and urges are telling us something important? I think of the engineering student, disciplining himself to study his equations when really he wants to play his guitar, because he "knows" music is not practical. If he has enough willpower, his musical talent will remain buried for a lifetime, but he will never be a very good engineer, or a happy one.

How much freer and happier we would feel, and how much more powerful we would be, if only we stopped struggling against the grain of our natural gifts and inclinations, stopped trying to be what we are not, and instead used willpower to stay true to an exciting and joyful life purpose.

Often we try to use willpower to improve ourselves: our diet, our bad habits, our selfishness, our temper. The fact is that any effort at self-improvement or change—including dietary change—relying mainly on willpower is destined to fail. If you resolve, "I will make myself do it," then you are fighting yourself. It means you are divided, that on some level you do not want to do it. Sooner or later, in a moment of weakness perhaps, or in a moment of self-forgetting, your true desires will express themselves as actions. The engineer's attention will wander, he will procrastinate, he will sabotage himself in a million little ways. The dieter will snack, cheat, make excuses, start again tomorrow. In a divided self, willpower is a puny thing.

The yogic approach to eating and diet is to bring oneself into wholeness, to illuminate and repair the self-division, to stop fighting oneself. Yoga, after all, means "union."

And even if you had an iron will, what a shame it would be for eating to become a regimen of self-denial! So many diets are defined by what you cannot eat. Who would not find the words "Yoga of Eating" intimidating? They seem to suggest a kind of discipline, purity, or austerity. It is significant that the very word "diet" in our culture has come to mean a diet of restriction—usually to lose weight. And so you may think that the Yoga of Eating is yet another chore, an incursion of self-denial into one of life's great pleasures.

Not so! Given the futility of coercive willpower, the Yoga of Eating offers an alternative: to align joyful, nurturing eating with the authentic needs of body and soul. To bring into alignment, into union, what you need and what you crave, what your body wants and what you actually eat. And, to integrate your diet with other life directions and your role in the world.

Healthy eating is not a matter of clamping down on unruly appetites. It is not a matter of the rational mind using its sophisticated nutritional knowledge to overrule a stupid body which craves foods that are bad for it. Second-guessing and ignoring the body is what has gotten us into this mess in the first place, and we will not get out of it by imposing on the body yet another set of dietary principles, no matter how new-and-improved they may be.

Whereas willpower implies pitting mind against body, in the Yoga of Eating we develop greater sensitivity to the body, greater sensitivity and trust. We stop seeing the body and its appetites as the enemy, but instead listen to the messages encoded in cravings, appetites, and tastes. As we develop trust in these messages, we discover subtler levels of sensitivity and greater unity of mind and body. The Yoga of Eating does not sacrifice pleasure; on the contrary it uncovers unimagined dimensions of it.

The Yoga of Eating requires courage. To abandon the habits of distrust, restriction, and denial; to emerge from the shadow of willpower and trust that the body is a friend that speaks truth; and to enact that truth even if it contradicts received beliefs about what is good and bad for you—this is no small step, but truly a leap of faith.

Chapter 2

Body and Soul

The body is not different from the soul, for it is a part of it; and both are a part of the Whole.
— Fariduddin Attar (trans. Idries Shah)

Man has no Body distinct from his Soul; for that call'd Body is a portion of Soul discern'd by the five Senses, the chief inlets of Soul in this age.
— William Blake

The idea that we live in something called "the environment" is utterly preposterous. . . . The world that environs us, that is around us, is also within us. We are made of it; we eat, drink, and breathe it; it is bone of our bone and flesh of our flesh.
— Wendell Berry

The ancient yogis considered eating to be a sacred act, in which one living part of nature absorbs and integrates another.

In our fast-food age, eating seems anything but sacred: a base physical act, sustenance for the body but certainly not the soul. Nourishment of the body and pleasure of the body hark to the animal part of ourselves, we think, while spirit is something much more refined.

7

We think this because our dominant scientific and religious cosmologies both hold matter to be separate from spirit and body separate from soul. Our science denies the latter categorically, while our religion sees the body as a vehicle or house for the soul, which animates it for awhile and then departs to another realm. The scientific view in its purest form was expressed by Richard Dawkins: "The universe we observe has precisely the properties we should expect if there is, at bottom, no design, no purpose, no evil and no good, nothing but blind, pitiless indifference."[1] According to this view, even if spirit exists, it has nothing to do with the world. As for the dominant religious view, it is that spirit is a separate and higher realm, and worldly things a distraction from spirituality. In other words, the world has almost nothing to do with spirit. Our science and our religion agree.

The distinction between body and soul mirrors another distinction, that between man and nature. Just as the soul inhabits the body, we see ourselves as inhabiting our environment: somehow separate from it in essence, though perhaps dependent on it for certain practical needs. Indeed, many people dream that we will one day leave the earth to colonize new planets, like a soul exiting the body upon death. In the meantime, believing ourselves to be above and beyond nature, we presume to be able to manage and improve on it—an idea that deeply influences the practice of medicine today.

It was not always thus. The distinction between man and nature probably began with the advent of agriculture, when we began to coax nature to provide food rather than gathering what was already there. The legend of Eden may encode a memory of this transition: originally everything was there for the taking, and we did not decide which plants and animals should grow and which should not. With agriculture, we partook of the Tree of the Knowledge of Good and Evil: crops and domestic animals were good, weeds and predators bad. We presumed to know better than nature what should and should not grow in a certain place.[2] And of course, to hold land away from its natural rest state requires work—expulsion from the garden into the world of toil.

The distinction between matter and spirit shares a similar origin, but only with the Scientific Revolution did it reach its logical conclusion. Before then, there was little distinction between God and Nature. The planets moved across the sky because God moved them. Animals lived because God animated them. God directed the weather. But starting with Galileo, Newton, and Descartes, the mysteries of nature succumbed to rational explanation, or so it seemed, and God became unnecessary, abstracted, banished to the heavenly realm. God was no longer a participant in nature; instead we had "natural science."

Before the Scientific Revolution, religion dealt with more than just the inner life of the spirit; it used to include cosmology, explanations for the way the world is. Science has usurped these functions, and religion has retreated before Science's program of explaining how the world works through experiment and reason. The realm of the spirit has thus come to mean the non-worldly.

Believing nature and the body to be mere matter, it is no surprise that our culture has, to a very great degree, separated religion out from material life, from life in the world.[3] Even the very word "spirituality" implies there are non-spiritual parts of life, denying that life itself is a spiritual endeavor. Dividing one's activities into spiritual and worldly reinforces the very fragmentation that the urge to spirituality seeks to remedy. Nonetheless, for lack of a better word and for the sake of expediency, throughout this book I will continue to speak of the spiritual.

The separation of body and spirit—and of man and nature—has become a poison to the world. Relegating spirit to an intangible, hypothetical corner of life renders the rest of life, life in the world, spiritually inconsequential. Because we see matter as essentially soulless, we view the body as profane and consider "worldly" to be an antonym of "holy." Without compunction then, we trash our planet and our bodies. Not holding them sacred, our abuse is limited only by practical concerns—and a very narrow, shortsighted practicality it is.

Not only is the desacralization of the body and physicality a poison to the world, it is a profound untruth as well. For the body is not the house of the spirit, it *is* the spirit taken physical form. And the world, too, is not the creation of divinity, it *is* divinity as presented to our senses. At least, that is an essential premise of this book. Issues of nurturance, self-trust, and mindfulness, even in the "basely physical" realm of food, reverberate with spiritual significance. That is because life in the world is a sacred journey, and matters of the flesh are potential vehicles for spiritual transformation.

According to this premise, the health crisis engulfing the modern world is a spiritual crisis, and a precious opportunity as well. Pain and illness in the body can illuminate what is important in life, and help us perceive the preciousness of life itself. Pain and illness bring us back to ourselves. Poor health can also be a message on many levels that something is not right. From the perspective of mechanistic science, the body is a faulty machine that needs an expert to repair it, an attitude analogous to the technological fix that ecologists criticize as a response to environmental problems. But if body and soul are not separate, then to heal the body at the deepest level is a work of the soul, and to listen to and learn from the body is to become closer to one's Self.[4]

The conventional body/spirit distinction is a temporary necessity, borne of their seeming separateness. As we explore the relationship between body and spirit, their underlying unity becomes increasingly apparent. If the body is in fact the soul made flesh, and not just its vehicle, then eating is indeed a spiritual matter. Eating defines a primal relationship between self and world, the receiving of sustenance and nurture. It is the tangible embodiment of the elemental relations of giving and taking. Through these relations, we can answer the questions, "How do I choose to be in the world?" and "How do I choose to be?"

Chapter 3

Birth and Nurturance

God created the child, that is, your wanting, so that it might cry out, so that milk might come.
— Jelaluddin Rumi

If we have had an incomplete experience of total, yielding, non-judgmental, unconditional love as babies and children, then our souls will yearn for it. It is a very deep need, a very deep hunger. Most of us had moments like this in childhood, special times with parents, a special relative . . . times in which we felt absolutely safe, that All was Well.

Sadly, at other times we had a different experience. We received affection when we were "good," punishment when we were "bad." At least sometimes, parental expressions of judgmentality made us feel we needed to be something other than what we were. Then, we became aware of messages from our peers, the media, school, the church, telling us, "You are not okay." Our peers taught us to conform by hiding or altering our true selves; the media created artificial needs, and promised happiness if only those needs could be fulfilled; the schools put work before play and instilled conditional self-esteem through grading; the church told us our natural thoughts and desires were sinful. In a thousand ways we were told, "It is *not* okay to be as you are: your body should look *this* way, your mind should not have *those* thoughts."

11

And so each of us, to a greater or lesser degree, picked up the habit of self-improvement. Self-improvement is an appealing but malignant idea, a poignant rejection of our innate goodness. It means that we have accepted and internalized those messages of deficiency, laziness, and sin. Sometimes people take up a strict diet in hopes of therefore being good, deserving, or pure, thus establishing a tendency to withhold from themselves what they really want or need. Even without this tendency, because our conventional dietary recommendations are a confusing mishmash of shoulds and shouldn'ts that seemingly have little to do with our desires as expressed in the body, a diet of self-improvement inevitably becomes a diet of self-denial.

But self-denial makes us crave nurturance all the more. When the experience of unconditional love and well-being has not been internalized, the soul seeks it externally—for example, from food. Food, an expression of Mother Nature's unconditional love and generosity, makes us feel nurtured and cared for. Food is the most primitive reminder that the world is good, that the world will provide.

All of us began life in this world with an experience of separation: expulsion from the womb. Before that came a nine-month eternity of Edenic paradise, where all our needs were effortlessly met. Then paradise grew constrictive; we grew up against the limits of the maternal environment. Finally this former Eden, paradise no longer, actively turned against us, expelling us with great force and finality into an utterly unfamiliar world. This journey is one of the great archetypes of the human psyche—the hero's journey, transcendence and rebirth. How does the story end? With a homecoming, a return to the One but at a higher level of consciousness. For the infant, it takes the form of the breast. The mother. Yes, the primal reconnection with the One comes from the experience of feeding. The universe has turned inside-out, but still it nourishes us. All will be well.[1]

The experience of eating thus relates on an absolutely fundamental level to our sense of security and comfort. In ideal circumstances the infant learns that the universe is fundamentally nurturing, that growth, change, and transcendence are safe, that there is no need to cling to the womb of familiar conditions when they have become restrictive, when it is time to move on. The infant is secure in the knowledge that the world provides. One can imagine what happens when, instead of the soft, warm breast, the first experience after the journey of birth is a cold, hard world where the infant is slapped, poked with needles, put into the solitude of the hospital nursery, subjected to a painful mutilation without anesthesia (if male), and fed from an impersonal bottle not according to his hunger, but to an arbitrary schedule. Actually, for many of us there is no need to "imagine" what would happen, because it *has* happened. The result is an unquenchable craving for security, an existential uneasiness in our relation to the world, a dread of growth and change, and a deeply troubled, unnatural relationship to food.

Remember that the need for nurturance is a genuine human need. To combat an unmet need with willpower is both foolish and futile. Only when we heal the wound of separation and accept and love ourselves without judgment does the need for external nurturance gradually wither away. One way this will manifest is in the diet. Without willpower, without denial or self-coercion, without the need for shoulds and shouldn'ts, the relationship with food will change.

Do not underestimate the need for nurturance in today's world. Even if you come from the bosom of a strong, loving family; even if you were spared the trauma of hospital birthing routines; even if you grew up in a tight-knit rural village away from the alienating effects of suburban living; even if no message "you are not okay as you are" ever reached your ears; even then, the need for nurturance may still be written into your very biochemistry. Anything that is born has experienced separation, and therefore, at the outset, has at least some need for external nurturance, the assurance of connection. Some of us are born much more emotionally needy than others. The karma we embody, as expressed through our genes and circumstances, usually limits to a very great degree the bio-physical changes we can make in one lifetime.

The hunger for external nurturance comes from deep beneath the conscious personality, and eases only when we begin to heal the fundamental fragmentation and self-separation that is its source.

Chapter 4

Food and Personality

Preach not to others what they should eat, but eat as becomes you, and be silent.
— Epictetus

People commonly assume that it is aspiration for enlightenment to abandon worldly ambitions and go to live in a hermitage in the mountains to clear the mind with the sound of waterfalls and the wind in the pines. But this cannot be called true aspiration for enlightenment. A scripture says, "Those who live in seclusion in mountains and forests and think that they are thus better than others cannot even attain happiness, let alone Buddahood."
— Muso Kokushi (trans. Thomas Cleary)

The body is like a lotus root, the mind is like the lotus blossom . . . . People today who want to avoid death forever and leave the ordinary world are imbeciles who do not understand the principle of the Tao.
— Wang Zhe (trans. Thomas Cleary)

Throughout history human beings have recognized a connection between food and spirituality. Most religions offer some set of dietary

15

rules: Judaism and Islam forbid pork; Hindus do not eat beef; some Buddhist and Christian sects maintain strict vegetarianism. Tribal cultures typically have foods that are taboo during certain times of the year, or for certain people, along with others that are considered sacred foods. In our secular age, religious dietary codes have given way to rational systems of food ethics. In particular, many people choose vegetarian or organic foods for ethical reasons: to avoid killing animals, destroying ecosystems, or using more than their share of the earth's natural resources.

The idea that some foods are higher or purer than others can be embedded in any of several paradigms. For example, we could rank foods according to the degree of consciousness we attribute to the being that died to become food. Accordingly, fruits are the highest, purest food because no killing is involved,[1] and plant foods are higher than animal foods because animals are (apparently) more conscious than plants. We could also rank foods according to their place in the food chain: foods lower on the food chain—that is, plant foods—are considered to represent a higher vibration than foods from animals, which are higher on the food chain. Another way of ranking foods is by the ecological and social effects of their production: the meat industry is deemed to cause the greatest harm, while to gather wild plants is said to be the least disruptive to the ecosystem. Many spiritual traditions hold that meat is denser, more congestive, or of lower vibrational frequency than plants; that green plants are higher than root vegetables; that fruits are highest of all. This hierarchy corresponds closely to the efficiency with which various foods convert sunlight into food energy. It takes far more sunlight to produce one calorie of meat than to produce one calorie of wheat. According to this paradigm, the highest, purest foods are algae and sprouts. Evidently, the ranking of various food types is more or less similar across all these paradigms.

For simplicity's sake, and for convenience of metaphor, I will use the much-ridiculed word "vibrations" to sum up the biochemical, ethical and spiritual quality of a food.

That each food has an associated vibration or density is a common concept in yoga and health-related literature, especially among

16

The Hierarchy of Vibrations—Dangerously Misleading

Density of Nutrition	
High	Fats, Organ Meats
↓	Meat
	Milk
	Grains & Legumes
	Roots
	Vegetables
Low	Fruits

Place on Food Chain	
Top	Meat
↓	
Bottom	Plant Foods

Degree of Consciousness of Beings Killed[7]	
High	Meat, Poultry, Fish
↓	Roots
	Leaves
	Grains
	Fruit
	Algae
Low	Milk[8]

Efficiency of Conversion of Sunlight to Food Energy	
Low	Beef
↓	Pork, Chicken
	Fish
	Milk
	Plant Foods
	Sprouts
High	Algae

groups that advocate strict vegetarianism or raw-foods diets. Generally, the lowest-vibration, densest food is considered to be meat, particularly red meat. Fish has a higher vibration; eggs and milk yet higher. Next come plant foods. Among the vegetables, root vegetables have lower vibrations, green leafy vegetables higher. Cooking food, it is said, reduces its vibrational level. Fruits have just about the highest vibrations, topped only perhaps by algae or sprouts. Above that we might find pure mineral water, then air and sunlight.

An assumption lurks within this ranking that more "evolved" people move on to foods of higher and higher vibrations. According to this point of view, the diet we choose reflects one's level of moral and spiritual development. Conversely, if you want to raise your own level, if you want to become cleaner, higher, purer, and *better*, you must raise your diet to that level. Meat eaters are morally and spiritually lower than pesco-vegetarians, who are lower than ovo-lacto-vegetarians, who are lower than strict vegans, who are lower than fruitarians. Raise the vibrational level of your food, and you will automatically raise the vibrational level of your self. Or so the thinking goes.

This assumption gains credence upon observation of monks, yogis, and other spiritual people who eat very extreme diets. Many Buddhist monks in Asia eat only one small, vegetable-and-rice meal a day. Legends of Taoist immortals, perfected people, have them subsisting on just the morning dew of the mountains, and there are similar accounts in India and the West of hermits and ascetics who eat nothing at all—yogis meditating in caves for months or years at a time, and the well-documented case of the Bavarian nun Therese Neumann, described in Paramahansa Yogananda's *Autobiography of a Yogi*. In America the Breatharian sect claims to live without even drinking water. Qigong practitioners sometimes report entering the *bigu* state (literally, "avoiding grains") in which they have no urge to eat food for weeks, months, or years on end, yet have normal energy levels and constant body weight.[4] "I want to be like them," people think. "I want to be pure. I want to enjoy super-health and super-vitality."

There is a fatal flaw in the logic of elevating oneself spiritually by elevating one's diet. The flaw is revealed in the following saying: "You cannot change one thing without changing everything." To be sustainable and health-giving, our diet must harmonize with our manner of being in the world.

Let us have another look at the idea that food is made up of vibrations. Shortly I will use the metaphor of vibration to explain the dynamics

18

of the diet-personality relationship; if you are put off by the New Agey connotations of the word, please understand that I am not here asserting "We are all made up of vibrations" as an absolute paradigm or ontology; nor is such an assertion necessary for the metaphor to be useful.

The hierarchy of vibrations, from meat to plants to fruit to sunlight, is dangerously simplistic. It is simplistic because each food represents not a single vibration, but a composite of many vibrations of varying frequency. It is dangerous because one is tempted to apply the same hierarchy to human beings, and conclude that some of us are higher, purer, and plain old *better* than others.

To see that each food represents not one but a composite of many vibrations, consider two heads of broccoli. Their vibrations represent the totality of their history and production, in addition to the innate nutritive characteristics of the plant species itself. Imagine that the first head of broccoli was produced in a huge industrial-type farm that relies on intensive use of groundwater, fossil fuels, pesticides, and chemical fertilizers. This farm engages in practices which poison the water and the soil; its produce is harvested by exploited migrant labor and trucked to supermarkets thousands of miles away. Broccoli with such a history will have very different vibrations from broccoli grown in an organic garden. One head of broccoli might be part of the destruction of the planet, another, part of its renewal. The two heads of broccoli share some vibrations in common, while others are distinct.

Perhaps all of these vibrations are biochemically encoded in the broccoli, perhaps not. Current scientific research certainly confirms that agriculture chemicals and depleted soil affect the makeup of a plant. But could a chemical analysis determine whether the laborer that picked the broccoli is treated fairly? This seems ridiculous. But it is a premise of this book that, whether biochemically or through some other mechanism, the entire history of a food is somehow bound up within it.

Now let us apply the metaphor of vibration to human beings. To imagine that the fathomless complexity of a human being could be reduced to a single frequency of vibration is a laughable conceit. Each of us

19

comprises a multitude of vibrations, some high and some low. Think of how differently you behave, acting from anger and acting from love. Different situations bring out a very different you. Haven't we all found ourselves, at different times, in the opposing roles of loyal friend and deceiver, sharer and cheater, sage and fool, healer and hurter? Different circumstances resonate uniquely with our being and bring out different aspects of our selves, different chords of our vibrational spectra. Nor are these different vibrations of our being haphazard notes; they are interwoven into a fantastically complex symphony in which each note resonates and harmonizes with the others to create the great themes of our lives.

You are a symphony of vibrations that encompasses every thought you think, everything you do, everything you eat, everything you are. Change any one thing, any one thought pattern, any dietary habit— change any one note in isolation—and you may introduce a dissonance. Nature abhors dissonance. Dissonance can be maintained only with effort, for Nature moves toward harmony and wholeness. Usually, the one thing you've changed reverts back to its original vibration. Something else can happen though: there is the possibility that all your other vibrations will shift to come into harmony with the one you've changed.

For example, suppose you have "poor posture" and decide to stop slouching. You find that you really don't know how to stand. You can try to just change your shoulders, but if you are attentive you find you must also adjust your chest, your pelvis, your neck, your entire stance. Either you can let your shoulders revert to their old position, reestablishing the old bodily theme, or your entire body will adopt a new pattern in harmony with not slouching. And not just your entire body, but your mind too must change—you find that certain negative mental and emotional states are simply not compatible with "standing tall." Either your posture reverts to a pattern compatible with, say, a defeatist mentality, or your mentality changes to a pattern compatible with a forthright and open posture.

Thus one might discover that there is no such thing as poor posture; that any posture is part of an integral way of being, reflecting and supporting who you are, an adaptation to your psychic circumstances and the

physical experiences arising therefrom. Some of these mind-body patterns, however, are much more painful and unhappy than others. The
same principles apply to diet.

Food, too, supports and harmonizes with our ways and means of
being in the world. Garlic, for instance, is shunned in Buddhist monastic
traditions because it has the reputation of "inflaming the passions": raw
garlic is said to stimulate anger and cooked garlic to stimulate sexual
desire. But we can also turn this around and say that raw garlic nurtures
and supports the angry personality; cooked garlic nurtures and supports a
sexually active body. The causality runs both ways. In the case of cooked
garlic, eating garlic and being sexually active comprise an integrated, self-
reinforcing state of being, while refraining from garlic and sex constitutes
a different, equally integrated state of being. To abstain from one and not
the other might cause disharmony.

Similarly, a person who has not fully internalized an experience of
the world as a nurturing place, a person who lacks inner nurturance, needs
comfort food to support that state of being. Someone like this who adopts
a vegan raw foods diet, perhaps to prove to herself that she is pure and
good, may be robbing herself of the nutritive elements required to exist in
such a mind state. She will not be eating in tune with the needs of body or
soul. The result is disharmony: chronic illness and joylessness accompanied by cravings that move deeper and deeper the longer they are denied.
Eventually she will die, or her diet will revert back into harmony with the
rest of her being.

It is now clear why imitating the diet of a holy person will not
make anyone holy. The diets of monks and saints are not usually a
practice, but simply the result of changing appetites. Therese Neumann
did not exert some monumental self-discipline to fight hunger pangs;
on the contrary, she simply did not feel hungry. If she used any willpower at all, it was simply to remind herself not to eat out of habit or
social convenience when she was not hungry. The same is true of
bigu qigong practitioners—they consider abstinence from food to be
an unimportant *side effect* of their practice. To genuinely emulate

these people . . . eat whatever you want whenever you want!

Remember the psychological origins of this idea of self-improvement: media messages that your body is ugly, a medical paradigm in which the body is unreliable, religious doctrines in which your natural thoughts are sinful, social affirmation and parental praise for behavior that isn't really you, and shaming for behavior that is. The notion that we must cleanse, purify, and spiritually elevate ourselves assumes that our current state is unclean, impure, and lowly. Another implicit assumption is that other people, who have not made changes to their diet, are unclean, impure, and lowly; callous, cruel, ignorant, or benighted. Not just in diet but in all areas of life, judgment of oneself always implies judgment of other people.

This state of being—judgmental, insecure, in need of nurturance—is not compatible with a high or pure diet.

Most people who thrive on extremely pure diets are somehow separate from this world, the marketplace, the world of dust. To live fully in the physical world, maybe we need a diet that is more grossly physical. The vibrational energies required by a hermit chanting the names of God all day may be very different from those required by us here in the thick of the human world. The menu of a monastery or spiritual retreat center nourishes a very different state of being than does the menu of a truck stop. If you adopt a monastic diet but not a monastic lifestyle, you will hunger for more substantial nourishment. On the other hand, if you gorge on hamburgers throughout a month-long Zen retreat, your diet will be a burden and soon become repugnant. If you wish to be deeply and fully involved in this world of physicality (and in my opinion there is plenty of useful and fun work to be done here), then perhaps you need the nourishment of this physical world as well.

By the same token, if you are about to depart from the world you may want to begin adopting a less physical, a less fleshly diet in preparation. The Tibetan teacher Sogyal Rinpoche tells of one of his great-aunts who, one month before her death, suddenly quit managing the household, stopped being busy with the world, stopped eating meat, and seemed to be in a constant state of meditation as she sang the sacred songs. Until then she had been an earthy, practical woman who enjoyed eating meat.

Some people don't wait until the end of life to begin detaching from the fleshly world. There is perhaps a time in the soul's journey to be apart from physicality, from carnality. Monks and people in spiritual retreat recognize this when they take vows of chastity and poverty, living without material complications. The disengagement from the world of the flesh goes beyond mere diet. As the former fruitarian Tom Billings discovered, a fruit-only diet forced him into a kind of social isolation, and the physical maladies he encountered, steps toward death, could be interpreted as a literal disengagement from the physical world.[5]

Just imagine how much greater the disengagement would be if you discovered you no longer needed to eat food at all. So many of our behaviors and ambitions are driven by the instinct for security, which is tied on a deep, biological level to food. Moreover, your experience would directly contradict the dominant scientific understanding of reality, and people with radically different beliefs from the majority often find themselves alienated. Inexorably, you would drift away from conventional work and conventional social life. It is very difficult to remain for a long time in consensus reality in one aspect of your life, and outside it in another. Eventually, something will give. Often that something is the diet. It is interesting and highly significant that when people claiming to practice total abstinence from food—or even a less extreme diet such as raw foods—bring their diet into the public view, they often begin to cheat on it. In 1983, most of the leadership of the breatharians in California resigned when their leader, Wiley Brooks, who claimed not to have eaten for 19 years, was caught sneaking into a hotel and ordering a chicken pie.[6] The obvious explanation is that he was a fraud from the very beginning. But another interpretation that equally fits the facts is that he only began to need food when he became involved in the world.

In my own experiment with a vegetarian diet emphasizing raw foods, I experienced a partial, though ragged, disengagement from the carnal world firsthand. On the one hand I lost much of my sex drive and found

23

it harder to engage in a normal social life. I became less energetic, my health less robust, as if my place in the world were more precarious. At the same time I became better able to invite and maintain altered states of consciousness, as if I were less tightly bound to the ordinary physical realm. My diet did not come easily or naturally to me, however. I was fighting myself the whole time, missing out on aspects of life I still wanted to experience. I was not at all ready to withdraw from the world of the flesh.

If disengagement from the physical world happens prematurely we will suffer and fight against it. Your soul knows when the time has come. If you are strongly involved in the world, for example bearing children, building your career, coming into your full human incarnation, then a denser, more fleshly diet or more earthy diet will support this. This is a generalization: the precise combination of food energies that supports you is as unique as you are.

Let us remember that to look down on carnality and elevate the non-material "life of the soul" again assumes that the body, and matter, is base, lowly, and profane—distinct from spirit. One's intersection with physicality has much to do with chance and fate. Some of us are cast to be householders, childbearers, controllers of material wealth, politicians, or to play other worldly roles, yet all of these harbor ethical dilemmas, a spiritual growth process, and the possibility to do Good Work. In a way it is much harder to be a good rich man than it is to be a good poor man. But if the world is to survive and humanity to realize its potential, we need people in the midst of materiality who use the things of the world wisely and well. It is only a temporary sojourn. Do not be in a hurry to get past it. There is important work to be done here.

A discrepancy between what we eat and who we are in the world generates a kind of tension, which is resolved either when the diet moves back in line with the person's incarnate role, or when the person's entire life changes to come into harmony with the new diet. Force, that is, will-power, can hold diet and being apart, but not forever. The tension will build, in the form of intense cravings, aversions, and, eventually, physical illness. The body speaks its message louder and louder trying to get what it needs, even as it does its best to function with those needs unfulfilled.

Chapter 5

The Karma of Food

You are what you eat.
> (Popular saying)

Wendell Berry has observed that eating is a political act, for it has consequences far transcending the individual. The way food is produced, processed, transported, and prepared has powerful effects on soil, plants, animals, and indeed the health of the planet itself, as well as on farmers, the rural economy, and all of society.

The idea of karma takes this observation a step further. Basically, the theory of karma says that in some way, all of these effects will come back to you. The theory of karma says that you yourself will experience the consequences of all your thoughts, words, and actions, including the eating of food. Accordingly, religions with explicit teachings of karma often advise against eating meat. The idea is that by eating meat, you are "eating" the suffering of the slain animal, and will eventually experience the same degree of suffering yourself.

In reality the theory of karma is more subtle than this. Causes and effects do not have a one-to-one correspondence; rather, causes combine in complex ways to create experience.[1] A detailed discussion of karma is beyond the scope of this book, but probably the soundest way to

27

understand and apply the theory of karma is to ask, "By this action, what am I saying 'yes' to?"

Let's consider a few examples. In the simplistic view of karma, generosity is rewarded by someone in the future being generous to you in return. But of course, giving with the expectation of eventual gain is not authentic generosity. By calculated giving, what are you really saying yes to? To a world where you have to look out for your interests, to make sure you get enough, and where receiving implies an obligation. In contrast, think of what you affirm by being generously charitable without thought of whether you can afford it. You are saying yes to a world in which there is plenty for everyone, to a universe of fundamental abundance. A truly generous person knows that there is plenty, acts as if there were plenty, and indeed lives in a world of plenty.

Similarly, by installing a sophisticated home security system, you may be affirming a reality that the world is not safe. By always being on your guard, you are reinforcing a reality that people are untrustworthy. By coldly eliminating the competition, you reinforce the reality that you live in a dog-eat-dog world. The mechanisms by which karmic effects manifest are not necessarily mysterious. Sometimes they are beyond current scientific understanding, but often they are not. For example, it is not so mysterious that we tend to trust people who are trusting of others.

It is an incorrect understanding of karma to say that if you have eaten a thousand chickens in this lifetime, you will experience violent death for a thousand lifetimes hence. By eating meat you are, however, saying yes to a certain version of reality, to a certain idea about the universe. The same applies to any food, of course, so for now let's go beyond meat and the mere fact of killing, to look into all the ramifications of dietary choice.

When you eat something, you eat everything that happened to make that food come into existence. You are affirming a certain version of the world.

For example, suppose you eat a banana from a South American plantation, located on destroyed rain forest land wrested violently from

28

indigenous tribes, who now labor at the plantation at starvation wages, using pesticides that pollute the ecosystem, shipped thousands of miles using polluting oil-fueled ships, by a company that puts small independent growers out of business through corrupt practices. By eating that banana, you ever so slightly reinforce this state of affairs, and make it part of your reality and your experience. You are saying yes to such a world.

Or suppose you eat chicken from a battery-raised hen, who suffered her whole life in a tiny, crowded, filthy cage, pumped full of hormones and antibiotics, painfully debeaked to prevent her from wounding her cellmates in her extreme stress . . . raised, basically, in Hell. Each time you eat such a chicken, you affirm the hellish suffering that brought it to you. Incrementally, bit by bit, you invite that experience into your reality.

Consider a very different scenario: a Native American hunter kills a deer with bow and arrow and eats the meat. The deer lived as a deer should live, a free life in harmony with nature, but one that ended in violence. The hunting is also sustainable and in harmony with nature. The hunter is therefore affirming a reality of wholeness and harmony, though with an occasional element of capricious violence thrown in. Interestingly, that is a fairly good characterization of Native American life before the arrival of the white man.

Now consider a squash purchased from a local organic farm. By buying locally, you strengthen community ties and ever so slightly weaken the hold of impersonal food corporations. You are saying yes to a world that treats soil, air, and water with respect, perhaps a world that respects all living beings. Even an organic farm, however, typically involves holding a piece of land away from its natural rest state; for example, preventing it from reverting to forest or prairie land. It is still a world in which we *work* to coax nature to provide. By eating that squash, you ever so slightly shape your reality and experience to conform to the set of conditions by which it came to you.

Ask yourself now, what kind of world are we saying yes to with our modern food system? When our food production system throws nature out of balance, is it any wonder that our lives too spiral out of balance? When our food system is based on the prolonged suffering of humans, animals, plants, and soil, is it any wonder that so many of us experience terrible physical suffering in our lives through chronic debilitating diseases? When anonymous strangers grow, process, ship, and prepare our food, is it any wonder that we often feel consumed by loneliness, estranged from the world? When we impose unnatural order on plants and animals through monocropping, genetic engineering, and so forth, is it any wonder that we too feel channeled and restricted, the natural flowering of our souls contorted and corralled into the unnatural, self-betraying mold society imposes?

Each piece of food is a repository of karma, a "symphony of vibrations" with high notes and low notes, passages euphonious and cacophonous. Is this symphony of vibrations in harmony with your own? Does it resonate with who you are now, and with who you would like to be? Does it nourish *you*? Are you happy with the reality you are saying yes to? With these questions, we arrive at the fundamental practices that define the Yoga of Eating.

Chapter 6

The Natural Breath

*The process of breathing, if we can begin to understand it in
relation to the whole of life, shows us the way to let go of the old and
open to the new.*
— Dennis Lewis, The Tao of Natural Breathing

*Real people of ancient times slept without dreams and awoke
without worries. Their food was not sweet, their breathing was very
deep.*
— Chuang-tze

As in many yogas, the Yoga of Eating employs breath both as tool
and metaphor. It is a tool, because breath is a powerful link between mind
and body; it is a bridge spanning various levels of one's being. It is a
metaphor, because the unnatural eating habits we impose upon our bodies
are similar in nature and origin to the unnatural patterns we impose upon
our breath.[1] Just as we are hurried eaters, we are hurried breathers. Just
as we've become numb to our bodies' authentic appetites for food, so
also have we lost touch with the natural rhythms of our breath. Recovering naturalness in breathing is a practice and a tool for recovering naturalness in eating. In both areas, we try to gain sensitivity to body messages,
and learn to trust those messages.

31

As you read the following discussion of the natural breath, try to draw parallels to attitudes about food and habits of choosing, sensing, and eating it.

Many people who have studied yoga, meditation, or martial arts have some idea of the benefits of deep, slow breathing. On a purely physiological level, deep breathing massages the internal organs, promotes lymph flow and venous blood return, and conserves energy. Deep breathing is also essential to Taoist and Yogic development of latent human capabilities through qigong and pranayama.[2] When people hear of these benefits and notice their own shallow, erratic breathing patterns, they understandably are moved to "improve" their breathing (just as one might "improve" one's diet) by learning to breathe more deeply. Unfortunately, to simply try to impose deep breathing on the body is futile, if not dangerous. Deep breathing is not something to "do"; it is something that should happen, something that should emerge.

Wouldn't it be terrible if atop all the things our culture tells us we should do and be, breathing itself were to become yet another chore, yet another thing to do right? We judge ourselves enough as it is. The idea of deep breathing is not to impose upon the breath, not to direct it or control it in any way; rather it is quite the opposite—to liberate the breath, to free it of the constraints already upon it. That is why the foundation of deep breathing is what I call natural breathing.

In fact, it is precisely this constant barrage of shoulds, shouldn'ts and can'ts that confines our breathing in the first place. We pinch and contort ourselves to fit into the ideal image society presents us, which makes it impossible to be at ease with who we are. Just to stand or sit at ease is something we rarely allow ourselves—always, we hold some physical, facial, or mental posture. Check right now: is your jaw relaxed? Are your lips soft? There is probably no one watching you at this moment, yet in all likelihood you are, out of habit, still presenting yourself. All of your postures, overt and subtle, all of your poses, project onto your breathing. That is why deep breathing is not attained through learning, but through unlearning. Similar logic applies to the diet.

The practice of deep breathing must begin with the practice of natural breathing. Even that is misleading. Let me say instead: Do not "practice" deep breathing. Let it instead be a side effect of natural breathing, something that emerges gradually with the successful practice of natural breathing; let it be an indicator that your practice is bearing fruit.

What an oppressive toil it would be, for every breath to meet some approved standard of deepness, to expect every breath to conform to some rule. And what a joy it is, to free your breath! The same joy of liberation applies to diet as well, and equally it requires a release of physical habits and mental habits such as belief systems.

A good teacher of yoga, martial arts, and for all I know, singing, calligraphy, painting, dancing, or cooking, can help you to rediscover your natural breath. Since each person holds himself in a unique way, the undoing of this holding is also intensely personal. Nonetheless, some general guidelines apply.

To begin, forget any preconceived ideas you have about what constitutes proper breathing, and form an intention to start from zero in rediscovering your breath. (We will revisit these ideas with diet.) Do not try to breathe deeply, or slowly, or to perform "belly breathing" or anything else. Without trying to change it, observe where your breath is going in your body, how your body expands and contracts with each breath. When you become familiar with the feeling of your breath, then begin to notice any ways in which you might be holding, constraining, or channeling it. Any kind of tensing in the stomach, ribs, or chest will likely restrict your breath, and you may find that tension in apparently unrelated parts of your body, such as your face, pelvis, or shoulders, has a strong effect on your breathing as well.

When you have totally relaxed around your breathing, it feels like the breath is breathing your body, not your body breathing the breath. You can practice natural breathing in any position. Just try to relax everything that you don't need to maintain that position.

33

Exercise 1: The Knee-Down Twist

The postures of Hatha Yoga are especially useful tools in liberating the breath. One of my favorites is the knee-down twist, which is especially useful for discovering how the breath inhabits the whole body. Lie on your right back, arms in T position. Bend your right leg and bring your right foot to rest atop the left knee. Then twist your torso, dropping the right knee toward the floor on your left, while turning the head to gaze to the right. It helps to scoot your left hip a little farther under your body. Usually it is advised to keep both shoulder blades on the ground, even if the knee is several inches up in the air.

Now relax around your breath, letting it deepen. Twists like this one can open up parts of your lungs that are ordinarily unused, so make sure to give your breath the time and space it needs to finish.

Notice how your whole body moves and expands with each breath. Many people find their left arm or right knee rising up on the inhalation and sinking on the exhalation. With attention and deepening relaxation you may discover subtle effects on practically every part of the body. Let the breath breathe you. Then after a minute or so, and before discomfort arises, gently bring your knee up, lie on your back, and after a few moments' rest, repeat starting on the left side.

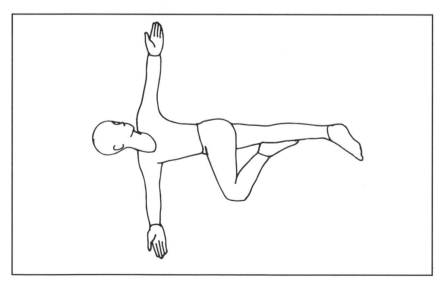

Exercise 2: Maha Mudra Breathing

This exercise is directed at using breath to communicate with your body.

(1) Sit down with your right leg stretched out in front of you and your left leg bent with the sole of the left foot against the inner right thigh.

(2) Adjust your right sitz bone slightly backward, so that when you bend forward you'll be coming down straight over the right leg.

(3) Lengthen your torso as you bend forward, grabbing your foot for leverage. If you can't reach your foot, loop a strap around your foot and hold onto that instead.

Now before you try to deepen the stretch at all, take a long, full inhalation. Do not force the breath to be deep, but *allow* it to be deep—give it the time and space to come into fullness. Then, on the exhalation, deepen the posture in one or more of the following ways:

- Lean forward, lengthening, as if you could bring your chest to your foot.
- Flex the foot, thereby lengthening the back of the leg.
- Bring the right knee closer to the ground.
- Press the tailbone and right buttock back toward the wall behind you.

From this new spot, again let the breath come in deeply. Notice how the entire body expands with the breath. If you are feeling a stretch in the back of your leg, it will probably intensify with the inhalation. If the inten-

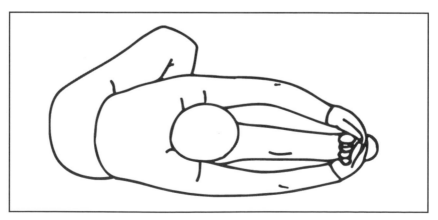

sity is so great that you feel you cannot take a full breath, then you are too far, and you should release a little on the exhalation. If it still feels okay, then on the next exhalation go a little deeper. In this way you are using the breath to ask your body, "Do you like this? Does this feel good? Do you want more or less?" Later we will query the body in the same way in the realm of food.

Really stay with the sensations and stay with the breath. You won't hear the answers if you don't pay attention. After you've explored this position for a few breaths, repeat with the left foot.

Exercise 3: Sun Breaths

Given that our physical holdings and postures are themselves habitual and unconscious, it is necessary to dig deeply if you hope to establish natural, deep breathing. The most formidable hurdle is chronic hurrying. Observe yourself sometime when you eat: do you hurry onto the next bite before the current bite is really finished? And breathing, do you hurry on to the next breath before the current breath is really finished?

Hurrying the breath is most noticeable in a moving series of postures, like Sun Breaths. Stand with your feet about 4-8 inches apart. On an inhalation, raise your arms through "T" position up above your head. On an exhalation, lower your arms back down to your sides.

As you continue this motion, notice whether you are leading with the motion, or leading with the breath. When motion leads breath, you begin the exhalation whenever the arms begin to move down. When they reach your sides, whether or not the exhalation is really finished, you begin the inhalation and raise the arms. Impelled by the movement, you are ending your breaths before they are really finished; you are hurrying the breath to keep pace with the motion. Or, perhaps you are artificially prolonging or holding the breath to keep it synchronized with your arms.

Instead of doing this, let breath lead motion. When the arms reach overhead, don't start bringing them down until the inhalation is complete and the exhalation starts of its own accord. This is more difficult than it sounds. Most of us in modern society have a habit of shallow, irregular breathing, or hurrying on to the next breath before the first is finished. Notice what happens at the transition between inhalation and exhalation. Is the breath finished, or do you just think it's time to move on? When we think, "That part's finished, time to move on," this is also an indication of what I call "success mentality" or "achievement mentality." If you think about it, success and achievement imply being finished with something. So try instead to sense whether there might be more breath coming in. Without forcing it in any way, give it space to come into fullness. Then, when the natural urge to exhale arises, let arms follow breath down to your sides.

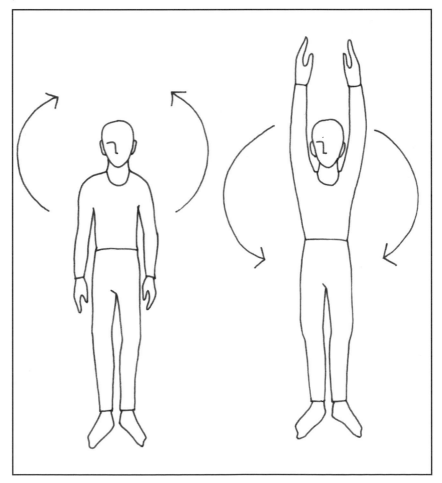

Exercise 4: The Tree

Rapid, shallow breathing is also a consequence of stress, of always preparing yourself for the next thing coming at you. If you work in a typical office, you know what I mean. It arises from a natural instinct of the body, which is getting ready for explosive action, getting ready for fight or flight. Draw back your fist as if to smack something, and notice what happens to your breath. If you are like most people, you hold your breath. This is a perfectly fine reaction, especially if you live in the forest and hear a crack of a twig behind you. Explosive action might save your life. But when the stimulus is chronic, the breath-holding becomes chronic too. A sense of urgency arises as you try to get your breaths in while you can. Eventually this continual holding and hurrying congeals in the muscles of the torso and the habit becomes ingrained.

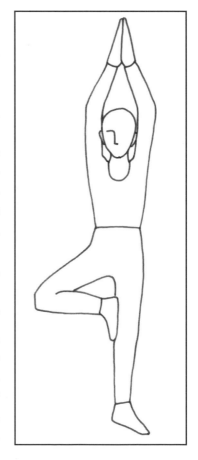

A good way to untie these knots is to put yourself under stress on purpose and practice natural breathing. A balancing posture like the Tree works nicely for this. Standing on one foot, place the other foot against the front of your hip, or against your inner thigh, or your calf (whatever is most comfortable, but try to keep your raised knee pointing sideways, in a plane with the rest of your body). Bring your hands into prayer position, then raise them up overhead. If this balance is easy for you to hold, then make it harder by closing your eyes. The idea is to make it difficult, perhaps even to generate some feelings of anxiety or frustration. Above all, keep the breath natural, even, and relaxed. Don't hold your breath. Let the breath flow, and take your time. Come into the posture slowly, over the course of several breaths.

If you fall, simply come into the posture again on a new breath. Hold the Tree until it becomes uncomfortable, then release gracefully with an exhalation, and repeat on the other foot.

The preceding exercises illustrate the combination of physical and mental habits that constrain the breath. Waiting and hurrying, anxiety and tension, pressure to succeed and fear of failure, all contribute to erratic, shallow, uncomfortable breathing. You cannot force yourself to breathe naturally without releasing your mental and emotional knots, without faith, acceptance, and serenity in your approach to life. You cannot compartmentalize yourself and see breath in isolation from every other aspect of your being. Here again I am talking about the "symphony of vibrations." Everything about you is related to everything else, and you cannot change one thing without changing everything.

While the deepest fundament of our selves reaches beyond even breath, the breath is nonetheless connected to our state of being far more intimately than most of what we ordinarily consider "mind." In other words, breath is much more real, much more fundamental than such things as thoughts and emotions. As such, breath is an excellent vehicle for accessing the deeper levels of the self. Like eating, breath can bring you face to face with things about yourself that might otherwise be inaccessible. It is true that you can calm the breath by calming the mind, but you can also calm the mind by calming the breath. The vehicle of breath can take you very, very deep.

Your natural breath is a treasure of the soul. It is a treasure far more reliable than just about anything else in this world, for as long as you are alive no power, no calamity, can take it away from you. So what happened to it? Where did it go? You breathed it as a child, but then when you became uncomfortable with who you were, when you accepted that you should be someone other than your natural self, your natural breath too became obscured. Know, though, that underneath all the impositions, holdings, and constraints, your natural breath still persists, a link to that child-like innocence now covered so thickly with all you have tried to be. Liberating your natural breath demands in the end that you liberate your natural self as well; equally, natural breathing is a pathway to self-liberation.

Chapter 7

The Central Practice

Drink your food and chew your beverages.
— M.K. Gandhi

The central practice of the Yoga of Eating could not be simpler: to fully experience and enjoy each bite of food. From this practice, all the other subsidiary practices of mindful eating are born.

Let us start at the core, with the physical acts of biting, chewing, and swallowing. To practice the Yoga of Eating it is necessary to devote your full attention to the sensations you feel as you eat—how else could you enjoy those sensations fully? Notice the aroma of the food before and after it enters your mouth. Notice its texture and temperature. Taste its combination of flavors on the tongue. You might find that different sensations register on different parts of the tongue and mouth. Start with these sensations, enjoying the deliciousness of the food, or noticing any unpleasant flavors or smells. You will probably find that the flavors continuously change as you chew. Starches, for example, begin to taste sweeter towards the end of mastication. The flavor of a food is not a momentary snapshot, but multidimensional, an experience extending through time. Eventually, when the urge to swallow naturally arises, pay attention to the feeling of the food moving down your esophagus, and to the response of your whole body.

Incomplete Experiencing

It may be hard to fully enjoy a bite of food, because in our society we are constantly moving on to the next thing before we're finished with the first. There is always something hanging over our heads, so many obligations, demands, and interruptions that we rarely have the luxury of devoting our full attention to any one thing.[1] Even as we do one thing, our minds have already jumped to the next.

This general habit is certainly projected onto our breathing, as we have seen. It is perhaps projected even more dramatically onto our eating. Next time you have a meal, watch how everyone shovels in a new bite of food before the first is fully chewed and swallowed. We cut short the experience of each bite in order to move on to a new one. Shoveling more food into an already full mouth corresponds to taking in a new breath before the old one is fully exhaled. Swallowing before food is fully tasted and chewed corresponds to exhaling before the inhalation is complete. This parallel to breathing is not merely incidental: hurrying and distraction in *any* area of life will eventually infect *all* areas of life. You may notice the same pattern in conversation—breaking in with your own speech before another's speech is finished; perhaps not even paying attention to the other's speech at all. You may see it in your work, in the form of distraction, your mind always moving on to what's next. Or it may show up as a general feeling of unease, a constant, nagging urgency that you cannot afford to fully devote yourself to the moment, that it isn't safe.[2]

Although the habit of incomplete chewing is an extension of our incomplete experiencing in all aspects of life, it also has a specific origin in the feeding of babies. You parents out there know what I mean. We shovel food into babies' mouths faster than they can chew and swallow. Even I do, despite realizing its harm. Babies eat very slowly and we have other demands on our time, and often the baby eats only a few bites before her attention is distracted by the nearest opportunity to make a huge mess. So, when you're on a roll and the baby is eating bite after bite, the tendency is to shovel it in quick before she changes her mind.

Perfunctory chewing and hurried swallowing rob body and soul of the benefits of food. Incomplete chewing hinders digestion. Digestion begins in the mouth (actually it begins before then, when the thought, sight, and smell of food stimulate digestive secretions). The saliva starts the process of chemical transformation of food into assimilable energy; for example, by breaking down starches into sugars. Meanwhile, the teeth mash the food into a pulp, maximizing the surface area for digestive juices to act on. When you hurry to swallow, the food goes down in larger chunks, the interior of which are less accessible to stomach secretions. Starches reach the stomach without having been predigested, and the cell walls of plant foods are still intact, rendering the nutrients inaccessible.

Despite its benefits, prolonged chewing (like deep breathing) should not be a goal in itself. To make it a goal turns eating into a chore, a discipline enforced by willpower. You may have heard to chew each bite twenty times, or forty times, or whatever. Such guidelines are of little value, because thorough chewing is properly a natural product of the Yoga of Eating, and not the essential practice. Again we make an analogy to breath: yoga exercises will foster deep breathing, but it is not forced; rather it is only a byproduct of patience and awareness in breathing, of easing into the freeing of your natural breath. Similarly, thorough chewing will happen naturally when you simply maximize your pleasure in eating.

Careful chewing should not be mechanical, but rather a consequence of the full, attentive enjoyment of food. This is great news. The Yoga of Eating calls for more eating pleasure, not less. If you adhere to a formula of chewing each bite X times, you'll chew some food far too long (like watermelon) and some, perhaps, not long enough. And without attention, you cannot access the subtle nutrients of flavor no matter how long you chew (more on this shortly).

Know What You are Eating

Earlier I observed how breathing is like another kind of eating. The converse is also true. Each bite is like a breath of air, and swallowing is like exhaling. A rhythm develops, and as with breathing, an unhurried, natural rhythm, in which you don't mentally or physically move on to the next bite while the first is still in your mouth, bestows energy, equanimity, and centeredness.

Continue in this way, bite by bite, through an entire meal, consciously choosing and enjoying each bite. Notice the sensations of hunger gradually giving way to the sensations of satiety. After the meal, feel the warmth in your body, the motion of your digestive organs at work, and the after-effects of what you've eaten.

Attentive eating uncovers unsuspected delights of flavor, unimagined subtleties of taste. You may find that foods you thought you liked don't really taste so good after all, while foods you thought bland harbor delicious subtle flavors you never noticed before.

Only by fully experiencing each bite of food does your body really know what it is eating. The body adapts in subtle ways to the symphony of vibrations, to the millions of biochemicals represented by each bite of food, mobilizing various digestive and metabolic resources, absorbing what is useful and eliminating what it not, coming into harmony with the food. But the body can only do this if it knows what it is getting, in large part through the instruments of the senses. Part of the body's reaction to this data will be messages that can tell you whether the food will benefit or harm it. You must pay attention to the food to really absorb it into the body for what it is.

In a sense, if your attention is elsewhere when you eat, you are not eating the *food* at all. The Vietnamese Buddhist monk Thich Nhat Hanh tells a story of a friend wolfing down tangerines while talking animatedly about something he was angry about, and points out that at that moment, he wasn't really eating the tangerines at all, he was eating the anger. So. . .

    — If you watch TV while you eat, you are eating the TV program.

    — If you read while you eat, you are eating the words.

    — If you eat when angry, you are eating the anger.

    — If you eat while absorbed by the scenery, you are eating the scenery.

    — If you talk a lot while you eat, you are eating your conversation.

This is to say that eating is a special time, even a sacred time, in which a person is in an especially absorptive state. While eating, the body is keyed to take in energy from the world. One is eating the entire experience of the meal, not just the physical food. The ambiance and emotional environment contribute to this experience, to the extent that they influence one's own state of mind.

To attain the full conscious enjoyment of eating, the best environment is probably that of silence. In company, a meal taken in attentive silence can be very intimate. It is said that good conversation is the best sauce for good food, but very often, words distract us from food, and food distracts us from conversation. Both words and food become not a way to intimacy, but a bypass. In silence a deeper sharing happens, for eating becomes a joint sacrament. Some of my students have reported profound experiences from sharing a meal in attentive silence, an intimacy of such sweetness it almost left them in tears. Alone, a deep and reverential sense of serenity, lightness, and vitality unfolds, and a close sense of connectedness to the all-providing universe. It is this connectedness that confirms eating as a path of Yoga.

Aesthetic Nutrition

In addition to grosser nutrients such as protein, fat, carbohydrates, vitamins, and so forth, food provides us with spiritual and aesthetic nutrition as well. Flavors and odors are themselves a kind of food, just as important as protein and vitamins. When you eat inattentively, you miss out on these subtle nutrients. When you become aesthetically malnourished in this way, your body, craving more flavors, drives you to eat more and more food, and foods with stronger and stronger flavors. To put it in simple terms, if you only taste a tenth of your food's flavor, then you need to eat ten times the quantity, or food with flavors ten times more powerful, to get the same aesthetic nourishment. Therefore we can infer a delicious irony: We overeat not because we enjoy food too much, but because we do not enjoy it enough!

It's not as if fully tasting food were a laborious chore; on the contrary, it multiplies the delight. So much of health and fitness these days involves self-denial. I urge you to practice the opposite. Fully enjoying each bite of food has a swift and dramatic effect on our dietary habits. You might find that your usual portion seems like an awful lot of food. Without willpower, you might find yourself eating far less than before. Without willpower, you will find yourself choosing (and preferring) healthier foods.

What happens when parents feed their children a diet of candy, hot dogs, chips, soda and other foods that dominate the senses? The first, direct effect is to damage their bodies and deprive them of nutrition. Even worse, the powerful flavors of these foods cause the tasting attention to become lazy, insensitive to more subtle, gentler flavors; you could say the palate has been spoiled.[3] Chewing becomes lazy as well, since the bulk of the flavor is obvious and immediate. The diet most American children eat actually renders them incapable of liking simple natural foods.

The subtle nutrients of flavor and taste also act synergistically with the grosser attributes of food. In an unprocessed, organic food, the flavors key in the body to precisely the nutrients it contains. Flavors are linked to nutrition—it is no coincidence that organically grown vegetables are both higher in vitamins and more flavorful, and that many potent foods have a strong and distinctive taste. The connection between flavor and nutrition is one reason why it is so important to eat whole foods, and why synthetic supplements normally bestow very little benefit. Additives and processing confuse the body by creating tastes not correlated with food's nutritive energies.

The link between flavor and nutrition is part of Nature's design. Odor is the main component of flavor, and it is primarily through volatile chemicals that plants communicate with each other and with their animal symbionts. For example, many plants are served by a single species of pollinating insect, which is attracted to their unique aromatic profile. Some plants can even generate odors that attract the natural enemies of insects feeding on them.[4] Food flavors, and one's likes and dislikes for them, are not accidental byproducts of a haphazard array of substances in food.

46

They are vectors of information, a biochemical language developed over millions of years of coevolution.

When you chew food thoroughly for pleasure, you get a deeper, fuller experience of the flavors from a given portion, fulfilling your need for sensory nourishment. Naturally, then, you will need less food, and simpler food. Not because of self-denial, but rather because you are already delighted with simple fare.

Chapter 8

Making It Practical

Beware lest you lose the substance by grasping at the shadow.
   — Aesop

The benefits of the Yoga of Eating come not from self-denial, but from uninhibited enjoyment of and delight in food. Nonetheless, the practice I have described may seem demanding and extreme. Meals, after all, are our main theater of social interaction. Who wants to spend every meal in silence? It would seem that the *Yoga* of Eating takes all the *fun* out of eating.

Before I address this issue, first let us ask: Why do we use meals for social interaction; for dates, for instance? One reason is that without distractions—such as a meal, a view, an activity, at least a cup of tea— interaction with other people gets uncomfortably intense. True intimacy develops under conditions of silence or joint creativity—and true intimacy is scary and uncomfortable. So, we use various means to keep intimacy at arm's length, interposing small talk, glances away, facial masks, insincere remarks, little jokes, changes of subject, sips of tea . . . or bites of food. Eating helps us maintain a comfortable distance from one another. Any time things get uncomfortable, you can escape into your food. Moreover, the acts and sensations of eating themselves dull one's awareness of other presences.

Of course, you can divide your attention while eating, keeping at least part of it consistently on the food, but then neither eating nor conversation will enjoy your full attention. Someone please tell me, what is so appealing about a meal that leaves you full of words and food, but satisfied by neither? To me, such a meal is merely entertaining. Often I walk away from it with no recollection of the topics discussed or the flavors of the meal. Sometimes we even have trouble remembering what dishes were served.

Therefore, in the full practice of the Yoga of Eating, when you eat, eat; when you talk, talk. Only with full attention can your body sense and assimilate the subtle nutritive energies of food. As for talking, the best conversationalists are those whose attention rarely wavers from the dialogue.

By now you might be getting ready to throw this book into the nearest trash can, for unless you are a monk, it is extremely inconvenient and probably impossible to eat all your meals in silence. Indeed, the full-blown practice of the Yoga of Eating entails a monastic sort of life. It is no coincidence that many monasteries in all traditions take their meals in silence. Nor is it coincidence that extremely pure diets, those consisting of just water, or air, or nothing at all, are normally only practiced by hermits and yogis in caves. In its fullest practice, the Yoga of Eating really is inconsistent with life in general society, life in the marketplace. It is impossible to change such an important part of life so radically without changing everything else along with it. Just imagine: how would your life change if forever more, you absolutely refused to compromise on your body's food choices, and absolutely insisted on taking all your meals in silence?

It is the same with any spiritual practice. The practice of radical honesty, the practice of seeing God in everyone you meet, the practice of repeating a mantra . . . unless you are prepared for your whole life to turn upside down, you'd best take them up gradually. If a practice diverges too far from where you are right now, it will create a tension that can only be resolved by giving up the practice, or by giving up everything that you are.

If your goals are not so radical, if all you want for now is better health and greater delight and mindfulness in eating, you need not practice attentive silence during every bite of every meal. In fact for most of you readers, those of you not living in a monastery or hermitage, I don't recommend doing that at all.

Let's not lose sight of the fundamental motivation. The goal of the Yoga of Eating is to bring greater enjoyment and delight into your life. Certainly, food is a great source of pleasure, but there are others as well. Good conversation, for example, is both a pleasure and an art form. If the conversation at a meal interests you more than the food, then by all means, devote your attention to the conversation. Never let the Yoga of Eating become a chore, a discipline. The purpose is more pleasure in your life, not less. And the premise is that the universe is fundamentally abundant, that riches are all around us. Pleasure awaits us, three times a day, just from food. It is there all the time. All we need do is say yes to it. The same goes for the pleasure of a natural breath, the sight of a plant or tree or human face, a friend's glad smile of recognition . . . the simple pleasures of being alive. They are yours for the taking! The default state of life is joy, from which we depart only temporarily unless we hold ourselves away by force. Stop holding yourself away from the riches of being, and you will relax into joy. Thus, the Yoga of Eating is practical! It is blindingly obvious.[1]

If you decide that taking all your meals in mindful silence isn't for you (it isn't for me!), then modify the Yoga of Eating so that it won't conflict with your other joys. Even a partial practice is very powerful. Here are some steps you can take to bring the benefits of the Yoga of Eating into a normal family life:

- Slow down your eating. Even if you are absorbed in good times and conversation, reserve a tiny part of your awareness to see that each bite is fully chewed and swallowed before the next one enters your mouth.

- Before all meals, observe a moment of silence or say a prayer of grace. This is actually a very powerful practice, and it takes less than a minute.

- Every day take one meal, perhaps breakfast, in silence, without the distraction of a newspaper or television. Devote that meal to just eating. Or if this is too difficult, devote just five minutes of one meal.

- At every meal, let the first bite you take from every dish be with perfect attentiveness.

- During lulls in the conversation, or when someone else is dominating a conversation you're not interested in, take the chance to patiently experience the pleasure of each mouthful.

Since the reality for most of us is that meals are a primary occasion for togetherness, silence is really not appropriate. And in fact, good conversation and the full appreciation of good food are not incompatible if we take our meals at a leisurely pace. In many parts of the world, a meal can last for several hours, and not only on special occasions. With plenty of time between courses and after the meal, conversation and eating need not be compressed into a single hurried span that allows only a superficial experience of either.

The good news is that when you practice attentive eating, even once a day or less, you progressively inculcate a habit of complete chewing and assimilation of nutritive energies. Eating becomes so enjoyable that it calls to you through the conversations and through the distractions. It is not willpower that draws you back to the eating sensations, but rather the sheer pleasure of the sensations themselves, which begins to overwhelm the allure of distractions. Just as meditation brings serenity and mindfulness to all of life, so also does a daily practice of the attentive eating infiltrate all your meals and all of your attitudes toward food.

When I present The Yoga of Eating and receive feedback on the experience of eating attentively, one of the most common complaints, particularly among college students, is "I just don't have enough time." For many people suffering the assault of busy modern lifestyles, it is perfectly true that life could not go on as normal if an extra hour or two a day were devoted to the attentive preparation and enjoyment of meals. If "practicality" to you means making no substantive changes, but squeezing something new into the cracks of your life, then indeed, the Yoga of Eating is not practical at all. There is no shortcut. As Chuang-tze put it, "I have heard of flying with wings; I have never heard of flying without wings." Even as tiny a change as a moment of silence before meals will reverberate throughout your life and cause a cascade of changes you cannot predict.

Learn to distrust diets that promise change without change. A switch of brands, pills, or supplements is unlikely to result in real improvements in health. This makes perfect sense if you accept my earlier observations about the connection between diet and "how you are in the world." Substantive changes in your eating habits of necessity accompany changes in your manner of being, and the mechanism for these changes is not necessarily mysterious. If nothing else, to fully enjoy food takes time and attention.

Let's decode what it means to say, "I'm too busy to cook and enjoy a good meal." It means that for one reason or another, you choose to spend your time otherwise. Most of us feel this choice to be a forced choice, and yearn to be free of the obligations that drive us scurrying from one urgent task to the next, multitasking when we can. When I ask acquaintances "How are you?" the most common response these days is "Busy," and it is not spoken in joyous tones. Many people, and certainly not just college students, feel oppressed by the accelerating treadmill of modern society: get up, feed the kids breakfast while getting ready for work, drive them to day care, work eight hours and probably more, do errands on the way home, drive kids to after-school activities, make dinner, finish the housework in the evenings, flop down exhausted in front of the television . . . the details differ but the pattern is the same, as is the feeling of oppression. At its core, the feeling of busy-ness is the feeling, "There is not enough time."

The alternative? To be not-busy is to live according to the belief "I have time to do what I want to do." Life may still be full, but the attitude is different; there is no feeling of compulsion. When busy, one often feels that every action is forced, every action is obligatory; that there is no time left for self, no time to create, no time to enjoy. The mentality of busy-ness already contains within it the belief that there is not enough time to enjoy food.

The realization of the deeper implications of busy-ness suggests a spiritual practice that I have found very powerful. Simply decide not to be busy. Affirm to yourself, "I have enough time." Immediately you will encounter a test of courage. For example, you might be engaged in some task when a visitor stops by your office. Instead of thinking, "Do I have time to chat with this person," think, "Do I wish to chat with this person?" It is hard because you are aware of deadlines, pressure. These are not fabrications. You might indeed lose your job, following this practice. You might indeed be late a lot, or never show up. Life becomes a series of choices—"What would I like to do now?"—rather than a series of obligations—"What must I do now?" This practice makes us aware of our power. The leap of faith required is huge though. Will everything still be okay if I just leave right now and go for a walk, go home and make a birthday cake? Will everything turn out all right? Will I still meet my deadlines? Will I live up to my office obligations? The leap of faith is huge, because in fact, maybe everything *won't* be okay in terms of the priorities encoded in your existing lifestyle. The faith is that from a higher perspective, everything will be okay.

How deeply to practice the Yoga of Eating is up to you. It depends on how much change you are willing to accept into your life. If you are suffering from a degenerative disease, you might be open to very profound change indeed. If you are completely happy with your physical and spiritual health, or are unwilling to give up any of the distractions and entertainments that accompany your meals, then you probably haven't even read this far. Please remember though, that even the most thorough change happens one choice at a time.

Remember also that while the pleasure of eating is a great gift, it is certainly not the ultimate joy in life. Nor is perfect health the highest goal. The Yoga of Eating may conflict, to some degree, with other spiritual values. For instance I would not try to impose silence on our young children at our family meals. Nor do I insist on eating only the foods my body truly desires when we share food as a family. Family harmony requires compromise sometimes, a gentle yielding love. The body is strong and the world generous. Both can accommodate error after error as they patiently await the time of healing.

Chapter 9

Discovering the Right Diet

As soon as you trust yourself, you will know how to live.
— Johann Wolfgang von Goethe

Be careful about reading health books. You may die of a misprint.
— Mark Twain

When people take responsibility for their own health and begin to investigate various dietary philosophies, they often end up very confused. There are hundreds of diets out there, each with its own compelling logic. There are diets based on religion, ethics, medical systems, anthropology, cleansing, the seasons, blood types. You can choose to be a vegetarian, a vegan, even a fruitarian; you can adopt a macrobiotic diet, a live foods diet, a Paleolithic diet; you can minimize fats, or carbohydrates, or proteins; you can base your diet on Chinese medicine or Ayurvedic medicine. Each of these systems has persuasive proponents who have benefited from them—often I find myself believing in whichever one I happen to be reading about!

The problem is, most of these systems are mutually contradictory. In fact there is hardly a food which is not proscribed in someone's dietary system. Which authority are we to believe?

Fortunately, the simple tool of fully enjoying each bite of food has the power to resolve any questions about food choices and diet. The only reliable authority, in the end, is your own body.

The body is wise, but in order to access this wisdom you need to communicate with it. First, by paying attention to your food as you eat, you let your body know what it is getting. (When your attention is elsewhere, when you eat mechanically, your body cannot sense and adapt to its food.) The second aspect of communication with the body is to listen for its responses to the food you give it.

As I observed earlier, when you taste and chew attentively you discover new flavors, some delightful, others distasteful. You might discover that some foods you like really don't taste so good after all. This is the beginning of the discovery of your body's messages to you about food. All that remains is to trust these messages.

Conscious, attentive eating is an infallible tool, but it requires considerable trust and courage. We are constantly barraged with messages from the media and, sad to say, from our medical establishment, that our bodies are not to be trusted, that we are near-helpless victims of their arbitrary breakdowns; that when our bodies do break down we need expert help to fix them; that foods harbor invisible, odorless enemies alongside the equally undetectable friends called vitamins; that we just need do as we're told, get 800 milligrams of this and 50 micrograms of that, avoid this and eat more of that, and meet minimum daily requirements of someone's list of essential nutrients. The disastrous state of public health puts the lie to orthodox nutritional standards, which are almost fulfilled by eating a single bowl of fortified cereal, yet many alternative diets are little better, relying on dogma over the ultimate authority of one's own body.

When we pay close attention to our food, we discover layer after layer of sensation, both in the mouth as we eat and in the body for hours afterward. As novices in the practice of the Yoga of Eating, perhaps we notice only the grosser sensations, the dominant primary flavors of food, and the most dramatic aftereffects. But as we continue the practice, our sensitivity quickly grows more acute. We find how different foods complement our emotional state, the time of day, the weather, and other foods. Eventually, our senses and sensations can tell us practically everything there is to know about a piece of food. All of its karmic associations are encoded within it, and accessible to our body via the senses. It may seem incredible, but it is possible to distinguish by taste alone a free range chicken and a factory farmed chicken, an organic banana and a conventional banana, a local apple and one shipped in from Oregon, a tomato picked by a loved one and a tomato picked by a stranger, a melon purchased and a melon given, a bowl of soup cooked by microwave, by electricity, and by gas. I say "by taste alone," though at this stage of sensitivity, taste becomes something more than taste; it becomes a window for the intuition. If all this seems improbable, consider French wine experts who can tell from a sip of wine the variety, region, and year of the grapes; even whether they grew in a sunny or shady location.

Often, the information we get from our bodies contradicts received beliefs about what is and isn't healthy, virtuous or right. Then our trust is put to the test. But the body is wise, and the rewards for trusting it great.

The body will first be attracted to foods that meet its most urgent needs. A starving body will hunger for anything, even rotting meat, to meet the raw need for calories. As the grosser needs are fulfilled, subtler appetites and aversions come to the fore. In my late twenties, after a prolonged period of near-veganism combined with a profound lack of inner nurturance, my body hungered deeply for animal foods, a hunger which at first I ashamedly denied. When I finally let myself eat meat I was suffused by intense waves of pleasure and well-being. Eventually, when I caught up with my body's pent-up need for animal protein and, especially, animal fat, I discovered that sometimes meat, particularly conventionally-raised chicken, had a certain stink to it; when I paid attention, it didn't taste so good after all.

When you listen to your body, it will guide you toward the diet that is right for you. This may conform closely to one of the common dietary philosophies, or it may not. When you notice such a pattern, books on diet can be a useful map to explore new food choices. You can also try one out for a while and see how it feels. Let's be realistic: if you have mistrusted or ignored your body's messages for decades, you cannot expect instant sensitivity to its needs. Sensitivity and trust must be built patiently. In beginning to practice the Yoga of Eating you will probably experience some dramatic revelations about food and nurturance, but you'll be confused sometimes too. Information on nutrition, based on one or another dietary philosophy, can be useful when you have no clear message from your body. Be careful though. I believe that some of the most fundamental tenets of orthodox nutrition (particularly regarding fats) are just plain wrong for most people; and any diet in the universe will be wrong for some people some of the time.

Whatever you do, please don't be dogmatic. Often, people feel wonderful on a special diet for a time, but then their needs change. Be especially careful with cleansing diets such as veganism, raw foods, or macrobiotics, which often bring excellent short-term results, but may not support the body's building phase. However persuasive the proponents of a dietary philosophy, however compelling its logic, never abdicate the ultimate authority of your own body.

The body's needs change. Often underneath one illness pattern lurk others, just waiting for you to gain enough health to express themselves. Think of your body as a vehicle that carries you from one life phase to another. If you stick dogmatically to any diet, even one that was perfect for one phase of life, you may deny your body the raw materials it needs to carry transformation forward.

Up until now I have consistently devalued willpower as an agent for dietary change. There is a useful role for willpower, however. (Remember, its proper function is "to extend wisdom and insight into times of imperfect clarity.") Practically speaking, no matter how hard you try, there will be many times when you are out of touch with the body's messages. Maybe you are in a hurry, or absorbed in a social event, or emotionally distraught. At such times, it is good to be prepared with dietary rules that you can discipline yourself to follow. You should formulate these rules in moments when body messages are clear. Make rules when you don't need rules, then apply them when you do. Eventually they become second nature. For example, I strictly avoid packaged foods containing hydrogenated oils, even though I cannot consistently sense the wrongness of such foods directly, especially when the hydrogenated oil content is low. In a moment of clarity this food ingredient tasted disgusting, so I made a rule for myself.

Do not write your rules in stone. Your "symphony of vibrations" is not sheet music, already defined and complete, it is a work in progress that evolves over time, with different melodies and themes weaving in and out from movement to movement. Sometimes you might go through a phase of life that is consonant with a dramatically different diet. For example you might go through a period of retreat or withdrawal prior to a major life transition, and be attracted to extremely simple plant foods and fasting. Then when you are ready to plunge back into life again, your body might call for something else. Do not be afraid to let go of a diet when it no longer serves you.

It is a good habit to question dietary rules, even those you devise yourself in a moment of clarity. Needs and tastes change. There are conditions under which the most noxious substances might be beneficial. Pure white sugar, for instance, was used in small quantities in ancient Japan and India as a medicine. Once in a while, attentively taste something you long ago decided was bad for you. This practice keeps a person honest and forestalls the slide into dietary dogmatism.

Chapter 10

Distinguishing Appetites from Cravings

You never know what is enough unless you know what is more than enough.
— William Blake

How can we trust our bodies to guide us in the area of diet, when so often the body seems to betray us with cravings for foods that make us uncomfortable or ill?

This happens because we use food for other purposes besides gustatory pleasure and bodily nourishment. Foremost among these is distraction. For example, when I've been taking care of a baby for hours and he is grumpy and clingy and constantly demanding, annoyance and frustration begin to rise and I'll sometimes have an urge to snack on something, not because I'm hungry but just to temporarily escape the situation, to distract myself. People working in offices often do the same, as do students studying for exams. Deep down, they don't want to do the task at hand, and the bag of potato chips sitting on the desk is a convenient, if temporary, escape. Are these people really hungry though? Are their bodies calling for sustenance? Of course not. Nor does this kind of distracted, mechanical eating allow one to really taste or enjoy the food.

Another abuse of food is its use as a substitute for other kinds of nourishment and pleasure that are lacking from our lives. Depressed people, for example, often end up eating constantly in an effort to stave off the feelings of depression. Eating is a primeval form of solace, of comfort, but no matter how much you eat it won't bring more love, nurturance, or acceptance into your life.

In childhood boys in particular are encouraged to eat heartily so they will grow up big and strong. Thus they are trained to eat for motives unrelated to hunger: to be a good boy, to be strong, or to be appreciated.[1] The real hunger is for unconditional acceptance, a hunger that food cannot ever meet.

To put an end to chronic overeating and snacking, again it is not enough to apply willpower or self-discipline. The snacking served a need—for distraction or solace perhaps—and if this need continues to go unmet, the snacking will resume or be replaced with another, even more harmful, addiction. For the snacking office worker or student, the problem really isn't the snacking, the problem is engaging in work not in harmony with the soul's work. When you are absorbed in an exciting creative task you have no desire to escape it by snacking. Escapism, distraction from life, is also often at the root of overeating at meals. After the meal it's back to life, and if you don't want to get back to life, you might want to prolong your meal. All that self-castigation and self-loathing when it comes to overeating is misapplied. You are not lazy and over-indulgent. The fundamental problem lies much deeper. In a way this is good news, because it means you are not so bad after all. Yet it also presents a challenge, because the solution to overeating is not so simple as getting a grip on yourself or exercising self-discipline; rather it requires genuine change, perhaps in your work, your relationships, your beliefs, or your environment. Overeating is an indication that there might be something wrong with your life, not that there is something intrinsically wrong with you.

Almost everything I have said so far about food cravings could also be said about drugs. Addicts know that willpower alone is powerless to stop their habit. We can thus interpret food cravings as an expression of an addiction. (Actually, anything that distracts or entertains is potentially addictive.) The addiction is not purely a psychological addiction: physiological mechanisms for addiction are known for many food additives.

Addictive foods include sugar, certain spices, vinegar, MSG, and caffeine. Insofar as a heavy meal (and a prolonged physiological fed-state) is associated with relaxation and deadening of mental activity, overeating may also be considered physically addictive in its own right.

Sometimes food cravings reflect the body's authentic need for a certain nutrient, but usually (especially in the case of junk food) the real need isn't for food at all. The food is just a substitute: sugar substituting for life's sweetness; MSG for excitement and zest for life; excessive food for nourishment in general. If you honestly listen to your body, you can distinguish between its genuine appetites and the psychological cravings we transfer to food.

It is not so hard, really, to make this discernment. Usually it is quite obvious. In the case of snacking and overeating, just ask yourself, "Am I hungry right now?" That's all there is to it, in sparkling simplicity. If you are not hungry, then you are not eating in response to a genuine appetite. The Taoist adage, "Eat when you are hungry, drink when you are thirsty, sleep when you are tired," with its reverence for nature and the body, embodies the essence of the Yoga of Eating.

Not sure whether you are hungry? Sometimes people have ignored their body's messages for so long that even such basic sensations as hunger become garbled and faint. Constantly snacking, they may never even feel true hunger. If this applies to you, I recommend erring on the side of not eating. Wait until you are sure that what you feel is hunger. Skipping a few snacks, or even a few meals, won't hurt you (unless, perhaps, you suffer from diabetes or severe hypoglycemia). When you are sure you are hungry, take the time to familiarize yourself with the physical and emotional aspects of that sensation, and then eat slowly and with attention.

In the case of cravings for specific foods, you need to somehow ask the body specifically whether you want that food. Sometimes it helps to verbalize the question: "Body, do you really want this?" (Yes, I know it sounds silly, but often it really works. Try it!) As part of your query, imagine the entire course of the eating experience, before, during, and especially after. What is the feeling of satisfaction like, physically? You will be able to sense where the desire is coming from.[2]

The breath is an invaluable tool in this querying of the body. When you feel a food craving, first try to locate it in your body. It might be in the belly, the solar plexus, the chest, the throat, the back of the mouth, or just about anywhere else. Then breathe into that feeling. Feel or imagine the breath actually coming into that spot. Next ask your body what it wants—the response will be a lot clearer carried on the breath.

This practice is especially useful in dealing with overeating at meals, when we find ourselves craving more food than the body needs. Remember in a previous chapter how, as we gradually deepened the Maha Mudra posture, we used the inhalation to monitor our bodies, to see how we were feeling, to feel out our proximity to the edge of our capability. The breath is a bridge between mind and body. So when you are eating and wonder whether you have had enough, simply pause for a moment with mouth empty and experience a deep, unhurried, complete breath. This automatically puts you into closer communication with your body, so that you will feel much more clearly whether there is a genuine body-desire to eat more. Overeating, gorging, is invariably accompanied by shallow breathing, especially incomplete inhalation.

Remember though, that a deep, unhurried breath is not a trick to stop you from eating more. It must be an honest question. Trust whatever result your body tells you.

You may very well decide to eat that cake, or that fourth helping; maybe because your body really needed it; maybe because the craving drowns out your communication with the body. Either way, once you've decided to eat, let that be okay! Just be sure to practice conscious sensing, enjoyment, and delight in each bite you take. By closely sensing that piece of cake, by becoming intimate with it, your body understands better what it is. Then next time the craving will be weaker, for knowing the cake intimately, your body will be less likely to accept is as a substitute for something else (see for example the chapter on sugar). To apply Blake's aphorism, it is necessary to really *know* what is more than enough, and in this case such knowledge can only come from a full and present experience of the sensations, thoughts, and emotions of overeating.

The instruction, "Let that be okay" can entail a dizzying leap of faith and bring a profound sense of liberation. We think: How could it possibly be okay to really let go? What if I stuff myself? What if I devour a whole box of chocolates? Two boxes! What if I lose all self-control? Ah, but that is exactly what I'm suggesting. Lose your self-control. Stop controlling, and start trusting a higher intelligence. It is okay, it is really okay. Your body is your friend and a wise friend at that. You will very likely find that when you sincerely give yourself permission to choose the foods you want, moderation comes effortlessly.[3] There need be no struggle. People seem to assume that "I'll eat as much as I want" equates to "I'll eat as much as I can," but this implies a prior assumption that we are by nature self-destructive, bestial, profligate. In fact, "as much as I can" is *more* than "as much as I want." The gorging, the bingeing, the incessant snacking, all of these are aspects of a war against ourselves, not our true selves unleashed. For such people, guilt is a sauce for all meals. I am sorry, but you'll have to do without that sauce if you hope to really perceive and respond to undistorted body messages. Instead, let your choice be okay, no matter how egregiously it violates your knowledge of nutrition and good diet and, with full attention, enjoy what there is to enjoy.

Be sure also to sense the aftereffects of your eating. Often when people overeat, they distract themselves from the discomfort by eating even more. So ubiquitous are the distractions and entertainments of modern life that we are typically oblivious to the damage our diets cause. The body might be complaining about the last can of soda, but you are already immersed in a television program. You never internalize the connection, "Soda makes me feel bad." If something you eat makes you uncomfortable afterward, it is imperative to patiently feel and experience that discomfort. That way the experience of eating becomes integrated with all its effects, not just the initial mouth-pleasure.

The most insidious means of distracting oneself from the aftereffects of unwise eating (and this applies to any addiction) is to promise,

"That was the last time," "Tomorrow I will go on a diet," or "Tomorrow I will eat sparingly." Soon we are thinking about a glorious tomorrow, not experiencing our present situation. It is understandable when the present situation is bloated, stuffed and somnolent that one would seek to escape it. However, by not experiencing those sensations one is doomed to repeat them, again and again, until they are integrated and understood as part and parcel of the entire experience of over-eating. If you are sincere about not repeating it, then you should make it less tolerable (by fully feeling the discomfort), not more tolerable (by pleasant fantasies about tomorrow). So recognize those insidious promises as distractions, nothing more and nothing less, and return to the present experience, uncomfortable though it may be.[4]

It is well known that as a culture we seek to avoid and deny pain, even the remotest discomfort. Narcotizing drugs, escapist technology, pharmaceutical painkillers, and ubiquitous distractions fragment and deaden our experience of life. When we have a headache we reach for the aspirin, when we have heartburn, for the antacid; when we have a worry or a sadness, we reach for the pleasant fantasy or memory. Thus we never fully integrate the effects of our actions with the actions themselves. There is a word for the unintegrated effects of actions: karma.

What is less well known is that we avoid the full experience of pleasure as well as pain. Fully experienced, even small pleasures can be very intense. Often celebration is an escape from this intensity, a moving on. Next time you feel that delicious pride of accomplishment, try just being with that. Very quickly the mind seeks to convert it into some new benefit, some new pleasure. Even in sexual intercourse, our culture emphasizes the orgasm, which is both the apex and the ending of pleasure. And in eating, we can hardly wait to move on to the next bite without really enjoying the first. Fully experiencing neither pain nor pleasure, we live fragmented, disconnected lives.

A conscious breath forges a reconnection among different fragments of our lives and selves. It brings one back to the here and now. During a meal, pausing for a breath breaks the habit of one-bite-after-another, activating witness consciousness. It weakens the enslaving hold of habit. Not only will you have a clearer message from your body, you will be more likely to heed that message. You don't need to promise yourself that you will heed the message; it happens effortlessly, or it doesn't. Pausing for a breath should not be conditional on an agenda of what or how much you think you should eat. Trust the power of the breath itself, and let the results fall where they may. The pressure is off. Remember, if you are using willpower, that means you are forcing yourself to do something that on some level you don't want to do. By coming back to awareness through the breath, you align your different levels of desire.

In Chapter One I wrote that the appropriate use of willpower is to remember ourselves, to bring the light of awareness into situations where we feel out of touch with ourselves. When you are about to stuff yourself with cake, the appropriate use of willpower lies not in forcing yourself to refrain but in remembering exactly how stuffing yourself feels, and listening to how your body feels right now. Only then is your decision to eat or not eat an informed one. An informed decision is more likely to be a wise decision.

Willpower thus applied brings one into closer self-alignment and greater unity, in contrast to fighting one's inner voice, and is therefore energizing rather than tiring. Sometimes, however, suppressing authentic appetites also brings a kind of temporary energy—think of the anorexic, flush with the victory of denying herself a meal. This is borrowed energy, but the temporary high it gives may mislead her into supposing she is resisting a damaging craving, becoming stronger, purer, more disciplined, *better*. Fortunately there is another test that unerringly distinguishes genuine appetites from the evil voices of false appetites (those that hunger for substitute nourishment and don't serve the real need). If it is a true, body-based appetite, then every time you deny it, it gets stronger. If it is a superficial craving, not serving a genuine need, then every time you resist it, it gets weaker. The same applies outside the arena of food. If your soul is calling for something, and you deny it, the call will wax in volume until life becomes unbearable. But if you resist a habit that distracts you from a joyful, creative purpose, its compulsion will diminish. The first time is always the hardest (but it may never be easy).

In communicating with the body, allow yourself to totally trust the results. Vow that you will accept your body's answer. Don't attempt to use this technique as a way of quelling or fighting the craving. Let go of any expectation that you will eat less or differently. We got where we are by not listening to and trusting the body. Any fundamental reversal of this state of affairs demands that we begin to listen to, trust and honor our bodies. For most of us, this demands far greater courage than to simply apply willpower. Willpower is a very small thing, really. It involves no risk, for it comes from who we already are. Surrendering, trusting, allowing change to happen without a program: that is something much greater.

Chapter 11

Loving the Body, Loving the Self

The attitude of "heroism" is based upon the assumption that we are bad, impure, that we are not worthy, are not ready for spiritual understanding. We must reform ourselves, be different from what we are . . . We become vegetarians and we become this and that. There are so many things to become. We think our path is spiritual because it is literally against the flow of what we used to be, but it is merely the way of false heroism, and the only one who is heroic in this way is ego.
— Chögyam Trungpa

When we hate and abuse the body and its earthly life and joy for Heaven's sake, what do we expect? That out of this life that we have presumed to despise and this world that we have presumed to destroy, we would somehow salvage a soul capable of eternal bliss? And what do we expect when with equal and opposite ingratitude, we try to make of the finite body an infinite reservoir of dispirited and meaningless pleasures?
— Wendell Berry

In our image-oriented culture it is often said we love our bodies too much. Again, the opposite is true—we do not love them nearly enough. We demand or wish them to be a certain way, we sacrifice them for other

71

goals, we adopt unnatural postures or even surgery to force them into the image of our vanity, we use drugs to extract pleasure from them. We ignore our bodies' true needs and enslave them to the indulgence of ego.

Typically, what love we do offer our bodies is a conditional love. Would the bodybuilder preening in front of the mirror still admire his body if it turned to flab? Would the beauty queen still love her face if it were disfigured? Love of a temporary, false, or idealized image of oneself is called vanity, and it betrays a rejection of the true self underneath. The so-called body worship of our society is really just image-worship, institutionalized vanity. True love of oneself (or another) does not require a person to measure up.

Neither does "health worship" reflect a sincere love of the body. There are people, most notably extreme adherents of various dietary philosophies or exercise regimens, who worship bodily health, seeing it as an indication of virtue, and disease as a sign of, or punishment for, some impurity of diet or practice.[1] According to this calculus, the healthy zealot of our scenario is superior to the sick people of the world. He is better than they are. He has found the True Gospel, and will not hesitate to proselytize. Very often (as with anyone who clings to pride) the result is humiliation—and what could be more humiliating to the health zealot than a serious illness?[2] But even if the health-worshipper never gets sick, what good does his health do? The body is our vehicle for living and acting in the world; it is meant to be used. There is more to health, to wholeness, than mere physical integrity. You have been incarnated as this body for a purpose, and to achieve it your body possesses tremendous strength, resilience, and resources.

Unfortunately, we often squander these resources pursuing trivial goals, fighting ourselves all the way. For example, in Hatha Yoga practice some people try always to push on to advanced postures, thereby proving themselves worthy and good. Conditioned by the judgmental "be a good girl" approach to child-rearing, and the conditional rewards of our educational system, they need to achieve something in order to give themselves license to feel good about themselves. The body, pushed faster and farther than it wants to go, does its best to comply. Your body serves you so faithfully that it will suffer injury just to comply with your wishes. If you hurt yourself in a deep backbend, don't get mad at your back. "I thought that's what you wanted me to do, " says your back, "and I had to break some things to do it. Aren't you happy?"

However you decide to use—or misuse—its strength and resources, the body does its best to oblige you. First it makes small sacrifices, minimizing the harm to its smooth functioning. It will happily sacrifice liver cells to protect you from the toxic effects of alcohol. The pancreas will exhaust itself to protect you against the effects of too much sugar. The body always chooses a lesser harm over a greater. When your intake of toxins exceeds the capacities of your body's cleansing mechanisms, it deposits them inside the body, in places where they will do the least immediate damage. Eventually, though, the body is overwhelmed. But even as it degenerates, even as whole organs and systems lose their ability to function, still the body fights on. All the while it sends you messages: "Please don't do this." And the loudest of these kindly messages we call pain.

For many of us it is hard to see pain as a kindly message, or the body as anything but a betrayer, an enemy, or, at best, a stranger—especially when you suffer chronic pain or a serious illness. It is a great leap of faith to trust your body, because from earliest childhood the media teaches you to loathe it by propagating idealized body images and concepts of beauty that no one can possibly measure up to. To this loathing, the dominant medical culture adds fear and distrust, for it sees the body as an errant machine, a traitor that breaks down and becomes sick because something is wrong with it.

In fact, the body always does its heroic best under the circumstances thrust upon it—either through our own ignorance, or through the environment we're born into. Moshe Feldenkrais, demonstrating his Feldenkrais Method on a woman with severe scoliosis, observed to his class, "It's not her fault! She has done the best she could! That right shoulder is the only way she survived! If she didn't get scoliosis, she would be dead!" From

73

conception onward, we have been subject to any number of physical and psychic toxins that challenged the healthy development of body and mind. Accordingly, our bodies have bent into various physical, chemical, and emotional contortions to accommodate these injuries.

Imagine a tree growing in rocky soil, next to a cliff, in the shade of bigger trees. To survive it must grow crooked to search out light and water. We wouldn't call it a bad tree for being crooked though; on the contrary, it is a wonderful tree, a heroic tree. Your body is the same, compensating and adapting as best it can to the barren, rocky soil and occluded sunlight of our modern society.

I'm not saying that if you are sick and tired you should learn to live with it. What I'm saying is that wherever you are right now physically, it is your body's wise response to the circumstances thrust upon it. Some of these may be beyond your immediate control—for example, pre-natal or early childhood trauma. But a lot of it may be just not listening to your body. Your body told you what it wanted, but you did not listen; you gave it harmful things, and your body did its best to adapt to them.

Like a young child, your body loves you totally and instinctively. Like a faithful dog, it stays loyal even when you kick and abuse it. What is the proper way to treat a trusting young child? With patience and un-conditional love. And that is also the proper way to treat your body.

As for the body, so also for your whole self. In this chapter I have distinguished between "you" and "your body," but as we have seen, this is a false distinction, though sometimes expedient. It is not as though your body were wise and "good" and the rest of you, fool-ish and "bad." Think again of the crooked tree, growing as best it can. Everything you are and everything you have done is a natural response to the conditions under which you live.[3] Even the ego, much-maligned among practitioners of Eastern spirituality, is an aspect of a funda-mentally unified and divine Self doing its job with perfect wisdom according to the circumstances thrust upon it. It is the ego's job to look out for your best interests, as the ego perceives them. The prob-lem is that the ego's perception of your best interests is often mistaken, even incoherent, ultimately leading to suffering without end.

Thus we see that the problem is not excessive self-love, but rather not enough of it. Self-love has a bad name in our culture. We are supposed to love other people more. We are supposed to be unselfish. I recommend the opposite: be more selfish. The hurts of the world come not from selfishness, but from a deluded view of what self-interest really is and what the self really is. To be effective in your selfishness requires a constant examination of the things you strive for. Are they really doing you any good? I'm telling you to take your selfishness seriously. Be selfish whole-heartedly. Elsewhere I have written, "Rational self-interest has become the dupe of our culture's priorities, so that it is neither rational, nor in our interest."[4] When we deeply examine what we ordinarily think of as selfishness, we find a sad delusion. I imagine a vast orchard, the trees laden with ripe fruit, and myself sitting in the middle of it, warily guarding a small pile of gnarled apples. True selfishness would not be to guard an even bigger pile even more carefully; it would be to stop worrying about the pile and open up to the abundance around me. Without such examination we remain in Hell forever, thinking that our new five-thousand-square-foot house didn't make us happy because what we really needed was ten thousand square feet. On the other hand, very often one must acquire a thing first in order to discover that it doesn't bring happiness after all. That is why even deluded selfishness is potentially a path to liberation, and why I urge you to be selfish as best as you are able. Believe it or not, to be genuinely selfish requires courage. When the investment in something is large enough, we dare not ask ourselves if it has made us happy for fear of the answer. After staying in studying throughout high school and college, missing all those fun times, then all those years of med school, and all those sleepless nights as an intern . . . after all those sacrifices, dare you admit that you hate being a doctor? To be selfish is no easy thing. How many of us, in our heart of hearts, are really good to ourselves?

The realm of food is a way to practice being good to yourself. Think of the greedy eater, eating more than his share, stuffing himself. That's an example of deluded self-interest, of not being good to oneself. The glutton really is getting more food. More more more! But he is hurting himself. If he were more selfish, if he made being good to himself his number one priority, maybe he wouldn't eat so much. It is an irony and a miracle. When you really decide to be good to yourself with food, the end result is a healthier diet, not a less healthy diet, even if the path to that diet might start out with an extra-large helping of ice cream!

To be good to yourself with food is such a simple thing. Your body tells you what it wants. Don't overcomplicate the matter.

The proper attitude toward one's self, with all its flaws, all its folly, all its selfishness and hurting of others, is one of pity, compassion, and understanding. Discipline is a crucial part of the spiritual path, but it arises out of a compassionate desire to prevent future suffering, not a hostile crusade to punish, correct, or improve oneself. It is a remembering, a gentle reminding.

It is the same discipline you might impose on a sweet and trusting child. Your body is like a child, not a stranger-child, but one that tells you its every need, if only in a very quiet voice. Be kind to yourself.

Chapter 12

Fasting

Salvation is not attained by fasting, neither wearing certain clothes, nor by flagellation. These are superstitions and hypocrisy. God made everything pure and holy, man need not consecrate them.
— Paracelsus

Sometimes when you listen closely to your body, the message you hear is a call not for food, but for fasting. You may observe this in animals, which abstain from food when sick, and in young children, who sometimes go days eating hardly anything at all (much to the consternation of their parents!).

The body naturally goes through cycles of building and cleansing. Digestion demands significant bodily resources, an expenditure of energy; when you stop eating, that energy turns toward housecleaning. Our ordinary lifestyles generate far more toxic waste in the body than it can efficiently expel, which keeps it in a perpetual state of unbalance. Fasting gives cells a chance to expel the built-up waste products of metabolism, cleanses the liver, kidneys, and colon, and restores balance to the body. When the imbalance is severe the body recommends a fast by killing the appetite, or enforces one, via nausea.

There are many books, ranging from the lunatic fringe almost to the mainstream, that advocate fasting as an integral part of health maintenance. Many people who try it become zealous advocates because the benefits can indeed be profound. For nearly every major disease there are stories of miraculous recoveries through fasting. Do a little research in this area and it becomes clear that fasting works *for many people*. It does not benefit every person in every situation however, despite dogma to the contrary. It is essential to let your body—and not a book or another person—be the authority. Moreover, there are as many methods or variations of fasting as there are advocates. Fasting is not a shortcut to health, not a magic formula, but another area that requires honesty and attention.

In my mid-twenties I became convinced of the benefits of fasting, and embarked on two water-only fasts of seven days' duration. Mustering all my willpower, I promised myself I'd persist through the seventh day no matter what. I completely disregarded the messages my body was sending me. I did not realize that because I have very low body fat and a high metabolism, a fast would be much more physically intense for me than for an average person. I am convinced that I did permanent damage to my body, if not in the first fast, then definitely in the second. I actually tried it a third time, but after the fourth day was suffering extreme weakness and lassitude—symptoms of starvation. Fortunately, I had enough sense to end the fast, but to this day I have a distinct body-memory of the feeling of starving. Many fasters report a radically different experience: they say they feel light and energetic. Of course there is discomfort, especially in the first 3-4 days as the tissues unload stored-up metabolic wastes into the bloodstream for elimination. You can expect headaches, tongue coatings, and light-headedness, but in a way these almost feel good. The sensations of cleansing are quite distinct from the feeling of starvation—I know because I've experienced both. It is therefore very important to be sensitive to exactly what your body is telling you: to stop when the body says stop, and not to override it with willpower. By the same token, when the body says "keep going" you may apply your willpower to fight the desire to escape the discomfort, physical and psychological.

In fact, the greatest challenges and benefits of fasting are psychospiritual. Fasting has dimensions far beyond what we usually label the physical, and it cleanses more than just the body. Because eating is such a convenient distraction, fasting puts us face to face with ourselves. A day without food seems to stretch ahead forever as the mind squirms, twists, and turns looking for an escape. Fasting is a meditation of the body; conversely, in the *Chuang-tze*, Confucius calls meditation "mental fasting."

Fasting is a spiritual endeavor in part because it eliminates one of our greatest distractions. To get the full benefit of fasting it is therefore important not to substitute some other distraction for eating. Do not try to make the time go faster by watching endless television. Do not try to make the time go faster at all. Do not kill the time. Instead, be with yourself. This is a time of coming inward—self time. Use it for yoga, meditation, or journaling. Stay in the moment, moment by moment. This is a sacred time.

In addition to eliminating an important distraction, fasting also brings one back to oneself simply because the associated sensations are often so intense. Be observant of all the reasons you give yourself for ending the fast, and try to distinguish real body messages from the excuses and rationalizations of mind. These escape rationalizations will be similar to the reasons you give yourself for withdrawing from any situation of prolonged intensity. By observing them you can learn about the things that make you quit. Some common ones are:

"Who says I can't? I'm just going to eat and no one is going to stop me!"

"That is enough. I deserve to stop now."

"I can't take it any more."

"I'll do it for real next time."

Each of these messages is a window onto one's self-imposed limitations. Watch them come and go, get to know them, and they will gradually lose their power (not just in fasting, but in any uncomfortable situation), because you will recognize them for what they are. Meanwhile, pay attention to the authentic messages of your body; in this case, hunger. When you feel a real hunger, not a desire for distraction or escape, that is the time to start eating again. Trust the body to tell you when the fast is over.

In its intensity fasting is very much like a spiritual retreat. It is no accident that most of the world's religious traditions have some practice of fasting: Lent in Christianity, Ramadan in Islam, Yom Kippur in Judaism, days of vegetarianism in Buddhism, and so forth. Many of history's great religious mystics, including Jesus, Rumi, and Buddha, also fasted as part of their spiritual training.

During a fast one experiences a distinctive clarity and lightness of being. All the senses wax sharper; everywhere you go you smell a symphony of odors. Sometimes you feel like you are walking on air, that your body is vibrating faster, as if it were in some higher plane of reality. One feels somehow separated from the world of flesh, rock, and soil.

Because of its associations with purification and cleansing, fasting is easily abused. Negative beliefs such as "I am dirty" and "I am impure," as well as the desire to be purer- and cleaner-than-thou, which stem from feelings of inferiority, may motivate one to cleanse the self's superficial levels—that is, the body as we understand it—without touching the deeper. When the fast is over, the spiritual need for nurturance is still there, combined with a feeling of finally deserving it. One thinks, "I have fasted, I did it, I accomplished it, therefore, finally, I am Good." Then, the reward: a return to old eating habits with a vengeance. It is impossible to maintain the tension between pure body and impure spirit indefinitely. Something must give, and usually it is the body, which returns to a state compatible with the mind.

The distinction between body and spirit is artificial, a conceptual convenience; yet we may provisionally say that the body is a map, a reflection, and an expression of the spirit. Inevitably, spiritual poisons will manifest in the body. It does no good to clean the body without doing any deeper spiritual work. On the other hand, because body and spirit are both facets of the same underlying unity, the body can be a vehicle for spiritual practice. It is an instrument for realizing unity.[1] Fasting is a spiritual practice, but only to the extent we do not escape the experience through some other distraction.

Similarly, when we purify the spirit, the body will naturally follow it toward purity. I have already discussed how we may gravitate to simpler diets when we realize inner joy and self-acceptance. Part of this process may be spontaneous fasting. All of a sudden the body rejects food, maybe overtly through vomiting, but more probably through a sharp abatement of the appetite. Trust the body when this happens, however long the state lasts. Trust your body to tell you when it needs food again.

When illness kills the appetite, trust that the body has a good reason not to eat. Although conventional medicine does not generally recognize it, fasting accelerates healing of many, if not most, illnesses, which is why physicians from Hippocrates onward have relied on fasting as a primary therapy. The issue is somewhat more complicated when serious illness results in prolonged suppression of the appetite. AIDS and cancer patients sometimes go to great lengths to stimulate their appetites, for fear they will waste away. In some cases this may be a legitimate concern. Someone with AIDS may indeed be able to prolong his life by forcing himself to eat.[2] I'm not sure. Personally, though, I trust my body so totally that if my body decided it were time to die, and shut down the appetite for food, I would stop eating. I trust my body's wisdom completely. However, this is a leap of faith that I cannot urge upon another person. Its rightness for me is self-evident, but that is for me. I am not *advising* anyone to do this, just pointing out that prolonging life may not be the ultimate good. Sometimes the body knows that it is time to die, and just gives up, shuts down. Animals do this sometimes when caught in a hopeless situation. Usually, though, the body wants to live, and by following the wisdom of its urgings, to eat or not to eat, you will live longer and better.

Finally, the body may also reject food, or certain kinds of food, during intense spiritual practice. It is as if by removing oneself from the world, one removes the need for food of the world. Just remember that when you return to worldly matters, your body will probably again require the sustenance of worldly food.

Aside from the atypical situations of illness and spiritual retreat, I think most people have days when they just do not feel hungry. Unfortunately we usually eat anyway, out of habit, for social reasons, because of medical doctrine based on distrust of the body, or just as an escape. In the practice of the Yoga of Eating, we assign paramount importance to these body signals, allying willpower and appetite against the forces of habit and escapism.

Chapter 13

Dieting and Self-Acceptance

All too often, when people hear about the Yoga of Eating it sparks a secret question: Will it help me lose weight?

Let me approach this question first by observing that it hints at distrust of and opposition toward the body. The body does not grow fat out of incompetence or error. Rather, weight gain is its optimal response to the physical and emotional conditions that surround it. If we force the body to lose fat without regard for the conditions underlying it, we are essentially demanding that the body be other than what it is. We are sacrificing its well-being, which the body instinctively strives for, for the sake of some image or notion of what the body should look like.

Such an attitude is inimical to the core precept of the Yoga of Eating, which is to honor and trust the body. We must be prepared to totally trust the body's messages even when they conflict with preconceived ideas about healthy eating. We must be prepared to trust the body's authentic hunger, whether that means eating more simply, or perhaps, eating richer, more nourishing foods.

It is true, however, that usually the Yoga of Eating lets one be satisfied with smaller quantities of food, since this food is experienced more fully and absorbed more completely into the body. Accordingly, one could easily pervert it into a technique for reducing caloric intake. You might think, "I'll chew and taste very thoroughly, and so I'll eat less—great!" The problem is that you have mortgaged your chewing and tasting to an ulterior goal, turning the Yoga of Eating into a means, a chore. Soon you'll become reluctant to practice it at all, because you are afraid you'll have to eat less. You will be fighting your appetites, not trusting them.

Even though obese people are almost certain to lose weight through the practices outlined in this book, ideally weight loss should not be a goal, or even a motivation. Such motivation is only necessary when we exert willpower. The Yoga of Eating does not primarily rely on willpower, but on delight in food. Your job is to listen to the body's needs and give it what it wants; the rest, be it weight gain or weight loss, is up to the body, which is of a higher order of intelligence than your waking consciousness.

Hold on! How could obesity be in any way wise, or in any way consistent with a person's well-being? The health dangers of being even moderately overweight are well-documented. "Cut the crap!" you might think, "I know I'd be much happier if I lost some weight. I'd be more energetic, more mobile, and healthier. What's wrong with that?" Yes. Being overweight is probably not part of your optimal pattern of being. However, your body shape *is* integral to your *current* pattern of being. It your body's proper and appropriate response to how you live and who you are.

When I urge you to trust the body's authentic hunger, please realize that this hunger is itself a response or adaptation to the conditions, both material and psychological, under which you live. Sometimes, the conditions to which obesity is a response are written into one's physiology on a genetic level. Even in traditional societies free of modern foods and food abuse, there is a very small proportion of obese people. Hence, your body shape might be so basic to who you are in this world, that it will not change in this lifetime.[1] You'll just have to accept it. Usually, though, obesity is a response to biographical circumstances which, though deeply buried in the unconscious mind, are in principle accessible to change. The Yoga of Eating is a doorway to uncovering these deeply buried circumstances. When you change your relationship to food, which is part of your way of being in the world, the adaptation of obesity may become unnecessary. Even so, the first step is, again, accepting yourself as you are.

It is instructive to consider that many obese people do not consume more food than the rest of us. Some even claim very persuasively to eat very little. Of course, excessive caloric intake can make you gain weight, but perhaps it is not the ultimate cause. If the body-soul has decided that obesity is the appropriate response to a given set of psychological, spiritual, and physical conditions, it will use whatever mechanisms are necessary to achieve this state. Increased appetite is one such mechanism, aversion to exercise is another, or maybe a reduction in basal metabolic rate. There exist compelling psychological theories of obesity. One is the phenomenon of "armoring," where the individual encases himself in fat (or sometimes muscle) in order to be insulated from the world. Obesity can also be a manifestation of an unconscious decision to be unattractive to the opposite sex. And in Chinese folk belief, moderate weight gain (especially in middle age) is associated with being prosperous and well-established in the world, as though good fortune were sticking to your bones.

Whatever the specifics, once the unconscious mind has decided to become obese it is sure to find a way. Similarly, when the circumstances to which obesity is a response are removed, the pounds melt away as if by magic. Such weight loss may or may not be attributable to a sharp curtailment of the appetite. Even when someone successfully "goes on a diet" and manages to keep the weight off, the diet's success probably rests on other life decisions. Another person may fail with an identical diet, and blame his inferior willpower, when really he was simply fighting himself: the dieting was not aligned with any other life changes. It is much better to let the body decide when it is time to go on a diet, and to trust that it is sure to do so when life circumstances support it.

In a previous chapter, "Distinguishing Appetites from Cravings," I observed just how great a leap of faith it is to "let it be okay," whatever your eating choices. Let it be okay, and fully experience it, and change will come naturally.[2] The same principle applies beyond eating, to all our thoughts, words, actions, and manners of being in the world. In our society this is especially difficult when it comes to bodily appearance. Among my college-age students, at least half the men and perhaps ninety percent of the women think there is something wrong about the way their bodies look and are. Often they find themselves angry at their bodies for being fat. Or, even worse, they blame their own weakness, imagining some character flaw—greed, laziness, etc.—is responsible for their fatness. It's either "Something is wrong with my body," or "Something is wrong with me."[3]

Because this mentality is so pervasive in our society, I will offer an alternative weight loss program in three steps, a program that respects and honors the body's way of being. As you'll see from the first step, I'm joking when I call it a weight-loss program, though such is a likely result. Whatever the result, the following description of the Yoga of Eating is especially directed at people who suffer from obesity or feel the need to lose weight.

Step 1: First, drop any wish or expectation that you will lose weight with this program. This is by far the most important step. (If you can't bring yourself to do it honestly, you can skip past this section.) Decide that you will honor and appreciate your body no matter what your weight is. Know that your body's shape is its wise response to circumstances that are probably beyond your understanding. Really let it be okay to be as you are. Don't hide any aspect of your appearance from yourself. Stand naked in front of a mirror and just notice all the criticisms and self-judgments. Don't attempt to quell them. Just let them run on, observing them. Underneath the criticisms though, let there grow a warm and wonderfilled appreciation for your body, which has done its best, its heroic best, under the circumstances thrust upon it. Think of all your body has undergone. . . yet here she or he is still alive, breathing, adapting. Allow a sense of grateful awe to develop. If your body condition causes you physical pain, let that add still more to your appreciation of the heroic effort your body is making. It is absolutely crucial that you begin this program with self-honesty and respect for your body.

Step 2: Apply the principles of choosing and eating food described in this book, particularly the middle chapters from "The Central Practice" to

"Loving the Body, Loving the Self." Focus on sincerely listening to the body's hunger. If you respect the body when it says, "Eat!" you will also be more likely to respect the body when it says, "Don't eat!" Respecting the body's messages will become a habit. Don't put conditions on your respect for your body.

Step 3: Now for your exercise program. Let's call it, "The Yoga of Exercise." Physical movement is properly a pleasure to the human body, but sadly in our culture it has become "exercise" or a "workout."[4] The goal of the Yoga of Exercise is to recover that pleasure. If exercise is a workout, one is tempted to skip it; if exercise is a pleasure, nothing can keep you away from it. Many former athletes give up exercising altogether because they think it doesn't count unless it is a workout (no pain, no gain). "I don't care for exercise," some people say, but what about fun physical movement? Pick a form of movement that you enjoy and that is easily accessible—walking is ideal for most people. Don't set any goals for speed or duration. Let the goal be just to do it, maybe even for one minute. But also leave the time open-ended so that you may go for more than one minute if you want. Trust your body. People lack exercise not because they don't enjoy walking, biking, dancing, or yoga; rather it is because they feel they don't have enough time. That is the mind talking, not the body. It's not even rational. No matter how busy you are, surely you have just one minute? Probably even five minutes. And no matter sick you are, surely there is some kind of movement that would be a joy to you. Walking very slowly, maybe, or some gentle stretches. Five minutes a day, even one minute a day, is far better than nothing at all; besides, if you enjoy it the five minutes tends to grow. Pleasure is a lot more reliable than willpower.

Step 4: That's it! If you started obese and sedentary, this simple practice is likely to make you lose weight. The Yoga of Eating (and of exercise) is far more reliable than conventional weight loss programs because it is based on enjoyment, not self-discipline. If you enjoy your diet and enjoy your exercise, why would you stray from them? All you need to is to remind yourself of what you like. That is the only willpower you need. Do that, and the changes will be permanent.

The above program is somewhat paradoxical, because it asks first that you turn your back on losing weight. But that is the whole key. By establishing a habit of self-trust, we are more likely to heed the body's calls for food (or abstinence from food), for exercise, and for appropriate rest. If you are sick or fat, you did not arrive there through bodily incompetence, and you will not permanently exit that state by continuing to treat the body as if it were an enemy.

I say permanently, because it is indeed possible to lose weight temporarily through self-coercion and self-denial. Usually it is possible (until willpower fails—see Chapter One) to keep the body below its natural weight by application of willpower. Even that doesn't always work—sometimes body weight remains stable or even increases despite sharply curtailed food intake. Moreover, it is a constant battle. Why live at war with yourself? Life need not be like that.

Your body weight is not just an accidental product of whatever diet you happen to adopt. It has deep connections to your manner of incarnation in the world. Unless these deeper conditions change, one's body is unlikely to change much either, except temporarily. This is something most dieters experience first-hand: as soon as the diet slackens, the body weight goes right back to what it was before. For some people, obesity is their lot in life, written into their very genes. For others it is an unavoidable phase, appearing or disappearing inexplicably as life goes on. But for most people, the deeper conditions to which the body wisely responds with obesity are accessible to conscious change.

Chapter 14

Fat and the Good

*And take your father and your households, and come unto me:
and I will give you the good of the land of Egypt, and ye shall eat the
fat of the land.*
— Genesis 45:18

Of all food elements, it is probably fat that inspires the most fear,
self-denial, and guilt in our society today. The antipathy toward fat within
the orthodox nutritional establishment and, increasingly, among the general public, comes very close to hysteria. "Demon fat" is how one popular
cookbook refers to it. We are told to reduce fat intake to below thirty
percent of total calories, or risk heart disease, strokes, obesity, and a host
of other ills.

Because our bodies tend to crave fatty foods, and because fatty
foods generally taste delicious to most people, one can only conclude that
the body is flawed. A healthy diet thus becomes a constant battle between our natural appetites and the received belief that fat is bad.

An historical study of language and diet tells us that our current anti-
fat hysteria is an anomaly. Older metaphors employing the word "fat"
typically connote abundance, plenty, and ease. "Living off the fat of the
land" implies a provident world; "the fat years" mean years of abundance. In Chinese the character for fat means fertile when describing
land, and munificent when describing a job or an opportunity. Notice that

89

these usages draw on the metaphor of a fatty piece of food. Fat is nourishing, enriching, life-supporting—a "rich" dessert is one with lots of butter. The negative metaphors associated with fat arise not from fat foods but from fat bodies. Interestingly, in Chinese the most common word for fat in describing a person, *pang*, is never used to describe a fat, *fei*, piece of meat, and I've been told this is true in other languages as well.

Today we conflate these two aspects of the word "fat," to the point where we believe that eating fat will make us grow fat. I will note in passing that the scientific evidence for this is ambiguous, especially when total calories are held constant. Most likely, it is carbohydrates, not fats, that tend to make us fat. Despite fairly constant levels of fat consumption, obesity in America has skyrocketed (according to some studies, by as much as 300 percent) over the last two decades. Various studies put the U.S. obesity rate at about twenty-five percent, while some three-fifths of Americans are said to be overweight.

Pre-modern diets put a high value on fat. In hunter-gatherer societies throughout the world, the fattest parts of the game, along with the organ meats, were the most highly prized, often being reserved for children. The !Kung of southern Africa wouldn't even bother to bring home a scrawny kill, but would just "eat the liver for strength" on the spot.[1] In rural China vegetables are served swimming in lard, if it is available, or peanut, soybean, or sesame oil—yet one very rarely sees obese people in China.

The near-universal esteem for fat in "primitive" societies is typically ascribed to their constant desperate struggle for enough calories to sustain life. Only, there was no such struggle. Except during rare natural or manmade calamities, food in pre-agricultural societies was abundant and easy to obtain. Even the !Kung, living in one of the world's harshest environments, only spent about 20 hours per week obtaining food.

So why our current terror of fat? Of course, many people try to cut back on fat, especially saturated fat, from concern over heart disease. It may surprise you to learn that the science behind the cholesterol-saturated fat-atherosclerosis connection is highly dubious, and many studies contradict it directly.[2] I am not a scientist, but I've read enough both of the conventional wisdom and dissident opinion to be convinced that any connection is very tenuous at best.

From the perspective of the Yoga of Eating this is a moot point, as we look to the body, and not nutritional scientists, as the final authority in our food choices. This is especially true in the case of fat, for two reasons. First, nutritional authorities disagree widely on the healthfulness of various types and quantities of fat. Secondly, the body's messages with regard to this food element are often especially clear. I recall an experience with coconut oil. I'd read that contrary to conventional views, coconut oil is very healthful for its plethora of medium-chain fatty acids. I purchased some high-quality coconut oil to try it out, and sure enough, my body responded gratefully—at first. Yet before long, eating moderate quantities every day, the very thought of the stuff disgusted me. My body was telling me I'd had enough. I've experienced the same repugnance when I've eaten large quantities of other fats too, particularly nuts.

Assuming that fat consumption causes neither obesity nor heart disease, then why has "low-fat" become nearly synonymous with "healthy"? Some cite economic forces at work in the pharmaceutical, food processing, and medical research industries. For a deeper answer, though, let us start with the ancient equation of fat with nurture, goodness, richness, and abundance.

When we have been born and raised believing our natural bodies flawed, our natural thoughts sinful, and our natural impulses lazy and indulgent, then we end up fighting ourselves in an effort at self-improvement. As children, perhaps, we made great efforts to "be a good boy" and to be "responsible," suppressing our real desires in order to live up to an external standard. Under such a regime, which starts, as I have pointed out, at birth, it is inevitable that pleasures become guilty pleasures. If you want something, it can't be good for you.

Accordingly, in education the exhilaration of curiosity has become the drudgery of study. The joy of creativity has become the yoke of work. The amateur, by definition one who does something for love, is denigrated in favor of the professional, who does something for money. Sex is perverted into an endless source of guilt and neurosis. The pleasure of physical activity—play—becomes the regimen of a workout. In all these things, we discipline ourselves and our children to withhold pleasure "for our own good." What a profound distrust of the self this reveals!

In our diets we do the same thing. Fat, traditionally associated with nurturance and abundance, has become the focus of our deep-rooted urge to self-denial, which is itself founded on self-rejection and a dearth of unconditional self-nurturance. The idea of withholding and denying pleasure for one's own good has a deep resonance in our culture, going back at least to Calvinism, Puritanism, and beyond to the idea of original sin. It is no surprise, then, that we have demonized fat on very ambivalent evidence. Our natural appetites are sinful, and fat is the Devil.

As I have written earlier, self-rejection increases the need for external nurturance all the more. No matter how strong your willpower, the body finds ways to get what it wants. People find it nearly impossible to stay on a very low-fat diet. They experience irresistible compulsions to cheat. You can make up for lots of missed fat with a couple pints of Ben & Jerry's ice cream!

Unfortunately, the fats available to meet these cravings are all too often highly processed oils, often partially hydrogenated, rancid, or damaged from repeated use in deep-frying vats. The health dangers of hydrogenated oils are well known, and the dangers of excessive quantities of other polyunsaturated vegetable oils are coming to light. These fats may satisfy the superficial levels of the body's craving for fat, but not nourish on a deeper level. How similar this is to the imitation pleasures on offer in our society, the packaged adventures, resort vacations, vicarious television thrills, spectator sports, and material consumerism that can temporarily deaden, but never truly satisfy, the longing to live fully and with gusto.

The current atmosphere of paranoia makes it very difficult to follow the body's wisdom when it comes to fats. The need for fat varies considerably from individual to individual, so listen carefully to your own body's messages, and trust those messages as much as you dare. Most of all, please do not hesitate to be good to yourself.

Chapter 15

Meat and the Life of the Flesh

To eat meat is to enact a profound transfer of energy and information, in which an animal loses its life to sustain the life of another. All eating is sacred, for it converts one part of nature into another, and because animals are (generally) more conscious than plants,[1] more highly organized, and a more highly evolved expression of the unfolding universal pattern, eating them has important spiritual implications.

Animal foods are the greatest expression of Mother Earth's loving nurturance. Like any good mother, Mother Earth will give everything she can to her children; she will give even of her own flesh and blood. And if it is demanded of her, she will give far past her capacity to sustain. There is a time in life, and in a soul's development, to be nurtured, to take from the mother. But a normal child will eventually mature and begin demanding less, begin giving back to his mother. Collectively, we are like spoiled, petulant, selfish children, taking and taking, demanding and demanding, wanting and grabbing, even as our mother lies dying from all we have taken. Of this frenzy of despoliation and plunder, the meat industry is one small but important aspect.

The meat industry as it stands today is one of the most prominent examples of collective human cruelty and callousness. I would like to emphasize, however, that I do not believe that meat farmers, or even meat company executives, are more evil, cruel, or immoral than other human beings. Their actions are strongly determined by economic forces and quite universal human mechanisms of rationalization. Most believe they have little choice but to farm the way they do, and most are barely making a living as it is. To a very great degree, people live the lives that are given them. To do otherwise is heroic, and while we might strive to inspire and support heroism in others, we cannot demand it or condemn its absence.

As I wrote earlier, by eating the products of our meat industry you are saying yes to Hell. The criticisms of the meat industry are probably familiar to many of you readers, but I'll review some of them anyway before moving on to some of the deeper principles regarding the eating of meat.

Meat animals are raised in horrific conditions of suffering, often confined to spaces so small they cannot turn around, crowded together amidst unimaginable filth. They are fed or injected growth hormones to bring them to market more quickly, and antibiotics to keep them alive. Their short and miserable lives start when they are prematurely torn away from their mothers, and end in slaughterhouses so hellish that even the workers suffer the highest accident rate of any industry. Feeding meat animals requires a huge input of grain and other plant protein which could feed far greater numbers of human beings than the meat does. Meat agribusiness consumes vast amounts of fossil fuel, which pollutes the air, and more importantly, consumes vast amounts of precious fresh water. It also poisons existing water with runoff from the animals' waste products, which contains traces of the antibiotics and pesticides in their diet. Wild ecosystems are destroyed through overgrazing, while the economics of the meat industry lays waste to family farmers and the rural economy. By eating conventionally raised meat you are saying yes to all this and bringing it into your reality.

Most of this suffering and destruction, however, is very distant from our everyday lives and therefore easy to ignore. People who cannot bear to swat a mosquito still happily munch hamburgers. This state of affairs is the natural consequence of treating so cavalierly an act as momentous as eating another animal.

Meat and the Life of the Flesh

The food industry—and the whole structure of our economy and society—separates us from the fact of killing. Anonymous strangers, who are themselves only incidentally connected to the animals, slaughter our meat, which is then butchered, processed, packaged, and transported by still other strangers. And more and more often, anonymous strangers even do our cooking. Thus it is easy to eat meat without thought of its origin.

Without any real connection to the animal, it is impossible to assimilate any but a tiny fraction of the energy in its meat. One is too far out of alignment with its symphony of vibrations. What is the alternative?

When the Native Americans ate meat, it was from animals they killed personally. They knew about death, digested death by being party to it. Moreover, they lived together with the animals in their natural habitat; they were part of the same web of energy and so shared many of the animals' vibrations. When they ate meat, it was in living recognition of how great a gift from Mother Earth they were accepting. They were saying yes to a reality of living in sustainable harmony with nature, albeit one in which occasional violent death was a fact of life.

Wild game taken in harmony with the ecosystem is a food far, far higher vibrationally than other meat, especially if the hunter herself is deeply attuned to the game's habitat. Any meat you kill personally will be far more compatible with your own vibrations than meat killed by anonymous strangers. Next best is meat killed by someone you know and love. Next, that killed by someone connected to you by something other than the utterly impersonal and distancing medium of money. As the connections grow more tenuous, it becomes harder to eat meat in full living awareness of the life it represents. It becomes less a sacred gift of Mother Nature's own body, and more . . . well, just a piece of meat.

The same goes for domestic meat. Farm animals can be raised compassionately as part of an organic farm; they can actually contribute to soil ecology, pest control, and resource circulation. Moreover, depending on the soil and climate, grazing animals on pasture is usually far less environmentally disruptive than horticulture depending on tillage. When you raise an animal yourself, you naturally become attuned to its energies. In fact you become fond of it, and the sadness you feel on killing it is actually part of the process of assimilating its energies.

What are you saying yes to when you eat such an animal? Some good things and some bad, probably, but certainly something very, very different from what you affirm by eating factory-farmed meat.

All food, and meat most of all, is a magnanimous expression of Mother Earth's loving nurturance. Do you have a need for nurturance? Paradoxically, it is often those of us who lack inner nurturance, who have low self-esteem, and who constantly criticize and compare themselves, who are likely to try to prove their goodness and deservingness by abstaining from meat. In taking physical form here on earth, all of us in varying ways embody a separation from God, from Source, from Spirit. This separation and its accompanying longing to return comes in many flavors—as many permutations as there are human beings on earth. One person might be shy and withdrawn, another territorial and domineering, but both are experiencing incompleteness, imperfection in self and world. Starting with milk from the mother's breast, food is a physical expression of connection to source, a reminder that the universe is in fact Good and that the world will provide. Therefore anyone who does not fully trust the innate providence of the universe will need, for a time, to avail themselves of the great compassionate gift of food. Of all food, meat is nature's most potent reassurance of connection and its most concentrated expression of nurturance. Depending on the unique patterns, themes, and intensities of your separation, you may have a genuine need to accept this, the highest of worldly gifts. It is a gift we should take with the utmost reverence and gratitude.

The neediness I speak of may not be traceable to events in this lifetime, but may be embodied in our physical constitution and body chemistry, the product of past life karma. Please don't think that a desire to eat meat reflects a deficiency of morals and character. As I explained in the chapter "Food and Personality," it may simply reflect a life fully involved in the world of the flesh, with its implications of sexuality, childbirth, and supporting a family. A life spent in solitary contemplation of the divine would not entail fleshly needs. I am not stating categorically that people living the life of the flesh absolutely need to eat meat; some, indeed, do not. In general, though, to sustain a state of being that is energetically involved in the world, and that is hale, hearty, and humorous, meat is necessary for most people.

You may choose to ignore your body's needs. That's okay! If you have a physical need for meat but nobly choose a vegan diet out of compassion, that is fine—as long as you can accept with equanimity and without resentment the physical degeneration that may follow. I have known quite a few vegans who have developed some kind of chronic disease or degenerative physical condition.[2] These include chronic fatigue syndrome, low energy, hypoglycemia, weak libido, anemia, multiple sclerosis, chronic yeast infections, asthma, and persistent cold-like symptoms. Physical degeneration is virtually assured if the motive for the diet is not entirely compassionate, but tainted with a kind of vanity—a factitious self-image of purity, superiority, or exculpation from the sins of industrial society. Self-righteousness and judgmentality indicate that vanity—love of an image, in this case the image of compassion—has (at least in part) supplanted compassion itself as the motive for eating a vegan diet.

Of course there are people who thrive on a vegan diet—most often people who are well-nourished in spirit, secure and generous, autonomous and nurturing of others. They do not take pride in their diet or derive self-esteem from it. They do not advertise it or urge it indiscriminately on others; they seldom even mention it. They are radiant people. But even these people usually do better with some amount of eggs, butter, milk, and cheese, unless they practice a very monastic lifestyle.

Let me hasten to add that while these positive qualities characterize the thriving vegan, they are by no means exclusive to vegans. It is foolish to attempt to draw direct links between someone's diet and their spiritual or moral condition. The relationship is not linear. It may be tempting to conclude that since meat is a denser form of nourishment and a more potent reminder of providence, that people who eat it are more separate from spirit. This conclusion ignores the fact that our means of feeding ourselves are legion. Food is just one form of the energy with which the universe abounds. Remember the "symphony of vibrations": people are a mixture of many different vibrations, some perhaps very high, others perhaps very low. Accordingly, their ideal nourishment comprises a unique mixture of different types of energy. Someone might eat a very pure diet, but be an emotional vampire. Another person might be very childish and greedy at the table, but open and giving in her relationships. Whenever I notice myself jumping to conclusions about a person's spiritual state based on superficial observations of their lifestyle, I like to remember two of the most enlightening presences I've ever had the privilege of knowing. One is a motorcycle mechanic. The other is a butcher.

I should also mention that some vegetarian activists argue, based on nutritional, anatomical, or anthropological grounds, that human beings are "not meant to eat meat." An exposition of these arguments is beyond the scope of this book. If valid, however, they would imply that any bodily appetite for meat is a false appetite, arising perhaps from social conditioning, and that you are deluding yourself if you believe your body is genuinely asking for meat. This is an extremely arrogant position, for it dismisses another person's sincerely felt sensations and says, based on dogmatic principles, that you know better than another person what that person really wants and feels. The central thesis of the Yoga of Eating is quite the opposite: that each person is the ultimate authority on his or her bodily requirements, and that the body will reveal its requirements given sufficient attention and trust.

Sometimes advocates of vegetarianism speak in terms of "moving down the food chain"—from animal toward plant foods, corresponding roughly toward moving toward the top of the vibrational hierarchy of foods described in the chapter "Food and Personality." But we can also see the food chain as a step-down transformer, which converts sunlight into denser and denser forms. Where you'd best place yourself on the food chain depends on what density of energy you need. A motor designed for six volts won't run twice as well on twelve. Of course a body is more adaptable than an electric motor—imagine a machine that can slowly modify itself to accept higher voltage—but nonetheless, an acute change in the energy input will cause dysfunction.

People who try to impose a vegetarian, and especially a vegan, diet upon themselves before the body is ready are attempting what is known in yoga as "premature transcendence," that is, to transcend the human realm without first becoming fully human. The tendency to do this is particularly strong among those not fully comfortable with themselves and their humanness. Remember, though, that the interests of body and soul are not opposed. Earlier in this book I have argued that the body and its appetites are not an enemy but an ally in the quest for health; equally, they are an ally in the quest for enlightenment.[3] It is not as Yeats said, that body must be "bruised to pleasure soul." Let us accept the body's natural appetites, however coarse and carnal, and trust that they will eventually take us toward a more enlightened state of being.[4]

Eventually more and more people will discover their interconnectedness with all other beings. They will discover—*not as a philosophical tenet, but as a visceral ever-present experience*—that they are not Alone. Realizing connectedness, they will no longer need to physically reaffirm it through consuming animals, or indeed, any form of life. Our destiny is to be vegetarians, and beyond that, to subsist on spontaneous universal energy.

It is a process that can be supported and honored, but never hurried or coerced. The anger and judgmentality of some vegan activists actually creates the opposite of what they intend, making people feel less safe, less supported, less nurtured and less cared for by the universe. Slogans such as "Friends don't let friends eat meat" reinforce separation, not union. Already too many people adopt vegetarianism to prove themselves good, to permit some self-love, to feel approved. All of these motives betray a paucity of inner nurturance.

Therefore if you would further the cause of vegetarianism, please, let other people know through word and deed that they are innately good, whole, and beautiful; that it is okay to be themselves, love themselves, and honor themselves without condition, reason, or justification. Prepare this, the soil of inner well-being, and compassion for other beings will sprout forth naturally, in eating and all activities of life. And yes, since ignorance renders compassion impotent, empower compassion with knowledge about the horrors of the meat industry and all that facilitates it. But do this kindly. Do this gently, patiently, and above all, humbly. The seeds of compassion will not bear fruit unless the soil is lovingly fertilized.

Chapter 16

Sugar's Sweetness

Refined sugar in all its forms (table sugar, fructose, sucrose, corn syrup, concentrated fruit juice, etc.) is arguably the most damaging factor in the standard American diet. Per-capita sugar consumption stands at nearly half a pound per day (between 40 and 50 teaspoons, depending on the study) and there is a close correlation between sugar consumption and the rise of chronic diseases over the last century in this and other countries. In addition to causing tooth decay, sugar upsets the body's endocrine balance, over-stimulating and eventually depleting the pancreas and other glands. Sugar strips calcium and other minerals from the body. These minerals are needed to metabolize the naked sugar, since its original accompanying minerals have been removed through the refining process. Sugar also causes fatigue and chronic low energy as the rapid rise in blood sugar provokes a massive secretion of insulin, followed by plummeting blood sugar afterward. Finally sugar is a major cause of obesity: once the liver has reached its capacity for storing glycogen, the body sequesters the energy from sugar elsewhere, as fat. The above is a simplified and incomplete account of the damage sugar causes the body.

Sugar offers a hollow sweetness that one can easily detect through careful, attentive eating. If you slowly chew and taste an oversweetened food, you'll probably find it phony and dishonest. Indeed, refined sugar cheats the body, promising a bonanza of nutrition that is not there.

Most people have at least a vague idea that sugar is unhealthy. Why, then, is our craving for this poison so compelling?

The root cause of sugar addiction is that we are out of touch with the sweetness of life itself. Our society, still cowering under the dour gaze of Puritanism, separates us from our essential core of sweetness and encourages constant self-criticism. The message behind every advertisement that shows us images of happy perfection is: "This is the way you should be. Are you not? Then buy our new car. Drink our soda." How often do I hear people say they want to be a better person? The person you are is just fine, if you would only let yourself be yourself.[1]

Closed off from the experience of sweetness in life, yet hungering for it to the depths of our souls, we turn to the imitation of this sweetness in sugary foods. Sugar does nothing to allay the essential longing, though; at most it temporarily distracts our attention from the soul's craving for sweetness. But where is the soul's sweetness to be found?

Babies are sweet. Intimacy is sweet. Love is sweet. Your innermost self is sweet. Think of the names we call our babies and our lovers, the people we know most intimately: honey, sugar, sweetie. True sweetness is found within. The experience of coming inward, coming back home, connecting with the divine, is one of ineffable sweetness. The term "sweet Jesus" is no accident!

The spiritual counterpart of physical sweetness is *intimacy*. Intimacy comes easily with babies, who are open and unthreatening, and with lovers (when there is genuine trust), and with close family. With all these people we can know sweetness. But we are meant for more than that. Outside the narrow realm of family (and with the decline of the extended family it has grown even narrower), we are closed off from one another, interacting on a very superficial level. How close do you feel to the people who make your clothes, your house, your possessions? How intimately do you know the people you buy things from? Intimacy comes from openness and long association. Today we rarely have either. In our tribal and village past, we knew each other intimately, having spent our lives together, and a stranger was a rare sight. Few people dare to be open and trusting of strangers or even casual acquaintances, and perhaps with good reason. Intimacy has hardly a chance to grow.

On a societal level, we may see sugary foods as solace in the face of the unremitting blandness and impersonal ugliness of the malls, freeways, parking lots, and windowless superstores that define modern life. We may see sugary foods as a primitive form of self-care under governments and corporations that seem not to care for us as individuals. We may see sugary foods as the last refuge of citizens-turned-consumers, stripped of their autonomy and stripped of the power to be good to themselves and each other in more meaningful ways. Tiny cogs, we seem, in a vast machine whose workings are beyond our control. In a disturbing world whose very infrastructure thwarts intimacy and has little time for beauty, who can blame us for turning to the nearest and most reliable substitute?

Yet, the powerlessness is an illusion. The truth is quite the opposite: You are powerful beyond imagining. Do you not feel powerful? Does your reason rebel at the very idea? That is because you have a mistaken idea of what "you" are. And because the self we operate from is self-limited, willful change (which comes from that self) is limited as well. It is like trying to lift weights while treading water.

Sugar consumption can destroy your health, but willpower alone cannot prevail against it unless you make an earnest decision to rediscover sweetness in your life. Rediscovering sweetness requires courage—the courage to give up things we think we need—as well as mindfulness or self-remembering to empower courage with the knowledge that those things are not so valuable after all. When we clear aside the clutter, the baseline of life is revealed: an omnipresent sweetness, a poignancy of connection that underlies life's sorrows as well as life's joys.

I am speaking of an opening of the heart, an opening to incredible riches that were here all along. Often such an opening happens when a death or serious trauma clarifies what's really important. We are so grateful then, and life so sweet. This opening, this acceptance of life's richness, is quite the opposite of the kind of self-denial that we might otherwise resort to in fighting the sugar habit. In fact, the habit of self-denial makes us crave nurturance all the more. (That's one reason why people who give up meat often turn to sugar as their comfort food, even though sugar is particularly damaging to vegetarians.)

Sugar is a shoddy counterfeit for the real sweetness of life. Often as children we were given "treats" as rewards, for being in some way "good." The word "dessert," in fact, means something that you deserve. When people try to limit sugar intake through willpower alone, they usually meet with some initial success. Feeling good about themselves, they are ready for their reward, for their dessert.

By the same token, sweets can be a way of telling yourself, "Yes, I *am* good, I *do* deserve!" Such a message is especially compelling to downtrodden people. Besides ignorance and poverty, perhaps this partly explains why poor people eat so much sweet junk food and suffer so much from obesity. People who affirm their deservingness of the good things in life through sweet foods are in fact using sugar as a kind of medicine. They are trying to make life hurt less. For a moment, at least, sweets make us feel less lonely. We are comforted. Do not condemn others for their dietary folly, when they, like us all, are merely seeking to avoid pain. Unfortunately, sugar is a palliative medicine only, as it does nothing to address the root causes of being downtrodden. No amount of sugar will fundamentally alter bitter circumstances or a sour attitude.

If sugar is a counterfeit for spiritual sweetness, then artificial sweeteners such as saccharin and aspartame are a counterfeit of a counterfeit. They represent a lie to the body, and reinforce an experience of the world in which appearance is bereft of substance.

Perhaps I am being unfair in calling sugar a counterfeit, because it can also be understood as merely the physical dimension of a cosmic principle or archetype: sweetness, comfort, pleasure. It is not through conditioning alone that sweet foods have become treats and desserts— were this connection wholly accidental, then I doubt sweet food would really work as a substitute for spiritual sweetness. Perhaps sweet foods are here to remind us and reaffirm that yes, life is sweet. Complete abstinence from sweets comes too close to Puritanical abstinence from all of life's pleasures; it can be part of a pattern of withholding from oneself the goodness and pleasure of life. Instead, let being good to yourself come first, and as your understanding deepens of what exactly it is to be good to oneself, you will find the craving for sugar diminish. Part of this deepening understanding comes from the full and careful experiencing of sweet foods, both as they are eaten and afterward.

So many things in the world today have robbed us of life's sweetness. The busy pace and constant noise of modern life robs us of the sweetness of "self time"—intimacy with self. Nor do we feel at liberty to really sit down and just *be* with friends or loved ones. The regime of self-criticism robs us again by making us not at ease with ourselves, and also, therefore, not at ease with others. When we are uneasy with ourselves, the fake fulfillment of consumerism and the ready escape of passive, asocial entertainment become irresistible. Ashamed of our own perceived ugliness, we wall ourselves off from others.[2] The economic and social structures of modernity build these walls even higher, by reducing our interactions to anonymous, superficial, or "professional" exchanges. And all these things, physical, social, and psychological, tend to cut us off from nature and thereby rob us of our primal connections to life, sky, wind, soil.

To quit the sugar habit, then, you must reclaim sweetness. Reclaim time in your life by reexamining the priorities that make you busy. Stop judging, measuring, criticizing, and comparing yourself; stop castigating yourself and wishing you were someone better, someone different. Instead, accept yourself as you are. The same goes for others: accept them, too, by looking for the goodness within. In all your interactions, try to penetrate to the human being behind the professional, behind the anonymous functionary. And perhaps most importantly, find ways to reconnect to nature. Even if it is for only half a minute, look at the clouds as if you had nothing else in the world to do. Touch a plant and feel its struggle in the poisonous air and tainted dirt of the city. Even small moments of intimacy can have a miraculous effect.

The sweetness of intimacy—with self, other, nature, or the divine—

is always there waiting for you. Sweetness can be yours without having to deserve it.

Chapter 17

The Yoga of Drinking

Many health and diet books advocate rules about drinking water: for example, that we should drink at least eight glasses a day, or that we should never drink water from thirty minutes before a meal to two hours after. Basically, these rules deny that thirst is a reliable indicator of the body's need for water. There are several studies that seem to support this. The Israeli army conducted tests of physical endurance under desert conditions in which one group of soldiers drank a certain amount of water at regular intervals, even before they were thirsty, while the other drank only when thirsty. The group that drank water before thirst struck outperformed the control group, seemingly proving that thirst develops only after the need for water becomes acute.

We are also told to "take plenty of fluids" when we have a cold or flu, even though a tall cool drink is usually the last thing we desire when we have a runny nose.[1]

Is the body's thirst mechanism faulty? Can we not trust the body in regulating our intake of that sacred elixir of life, water?

Just as with food, the problem here is not that the body is giving us wrong messages, but that we are insensitive to its real messages. What most people call thirst is a fairly extreme stage of the body's call for water. The beginnings of thirst are really quite delicate, and they start long before the throat and mouth become dry. The Israeli soldiers in the study were probably not sensitive to the subtler levels of thirst; that's perhaps one reason why they didn't get the water they needed.[2]

Drinking eight glasses of water a day is probably helpful to people who are chronically dehydrated due to over-processed diets and insensitivity to subtle thirst. The advice probably does more good than harm to the average American. Nonetheless, it could also lead to over-consumption of water, which is harmful to the body's electrolyte balance and other processes. Chinese medicine recognizes over-consumption of water, particularly cold water, as an indubitable cause of disease.

The marvelous mechanism of thirst is precisely calibrated to maintain the body in an exquisite state of balance. To distrust and reject it is folly. Just as the hungers of the body can guide us to healthy foods, so also we should learn to fully listen to and trust this important body message.

It's not easy, because most of us live in profound ignorance of our bodies. Until the body demands attention loudly (through pain, hunger, acute thirst, etc.), we ignore it, exploiting it for maximum pleasure, work, and benefit, squeezing out as much as possible. Oblivious to its messages, even when we finally decide to be good to our bodies, we hardly know how. Always some distraction occupies the mind, so that we rarely pause and listen to the body. Yet pausing and listening, and not some decision to drink X glasses of water a day, is the only way to hear the call of thirst.

First, learn to identify your subtler levels of thirst. Tune in to your body and ask whether it would like water. Imagine the sensation of drinking. Picture the liquid going down your throat. Would it be a pleasure to drink? If so, then drink. If not, then wait. How could it be any simpler? Yet even such simplicity demands patience and trust.

What a relief and a joy it is, never to coerce the body to drink, and to make every mouthful a refreshing pleasure!

Just as with food, when you drink water your senses can tell you much about its quality and wholesomeness. Water usually has a taste, which is what cues the body to respond appropriately to absorb and respond to it.[3] If the thirst is small, then drink your water in modest sips. Your body will then know how much it is getting, so it can tell you when to stop. If you are very thirsty, go ahead and drink faster, because it really feels good! Then when the edge of the thirst is slaked, drink more slowly and attentively. Always listen to your body's desires to drink and to stop— this is the Yoga of Drinking.

The principle of listening to and trusting your thirst also applies when you are sick. Do not believe on someone else's authority that you should always drink lots of water when you have a cold. In traditional Chinese medicine, some colds are linked to the body's expulsion of harmful "cold" and "damp" elements; accordingly, drinking lots of cool water will prolong the cold. You don't need an expert Chinese diagnostician to figure this out though; simply pay attention to your body's messages. Your body will tell you what it needs. Trust it. Bodies do not break down from their own incompetence; they break down because they are mistreated.[4, 5] Healing, then, is not the fixing of a miscreant body, but rather a removal of the impediments to self-healing, an unleashing of the body's natural self-repair systems.

Whether in sickness or in health, the body communicates its need for water. There are no rules to remember, no techniques to practice. Simply learn to understand the body's messages, and ease into joyful cooperation with your body.

What if you are thirsty at mealtime? What they say is generally true: drinking too much water (especially icewater) with food can indeed interfere with digestion. The body is wise, though, and knows enough to take this into account when demanding water. If you are well-hydrated beforehand and eat simple, whole foods, you probably won't be thirsty in the first place. It is only when we consume over-salted, over-sweetened, and over-processed foods in excessive quantities that thirst arises so quickly. If you ignore this thirst and maintain the same eating habits, the damage from dehydration will be more serious than that from dilution of digestive juices. (Indeed, dehydration can hamper the metabolic processes that accompany digestion and assimilation.) If you listen to your body's natural appetites you won't have the problem of thirst at mealtimes, but if you do eat a particularly dehydrating meal, or if you come to the dinner table thirsty after a hot day in the sun, then by all means trust the body's call for water. Besides, in my experience a little room-temperature water doesn't hurt digestion at all, though this might be different for your body. The main thing to avoid is washing down food with beverages, which are a poor substitute indeed for thorough ensalivation.

So far I have referred to water as the primary thirst-quencher. It is instructive to learn that some traditional cultures rarely drank water. In China, for example, to this day you never see water served with meals—the beverages are soup, tea, or a fermented beverage such as beer. Warm beverages are much gentler on the digestion than cold ones, while some soups and fermented beverages actually aid digestion. However, the sad fact is that most of these healthful drinks have disappeared from the American culinary scene. For most people reading this book, the best readily available beverage for quenching thirst is probably water; nonetheless, I will say a few things about some other drinks.

Beverages other than water combine the properties of foods and drinks, satisfying both hunger and thirst. **Fruit juices** are highly concentrated foods that need to be taken very slowly, chewed almost, in order for the body to come to terms with their full essence. From the body's point of view, they are also highly processed (since they require no chewing). A quart of orange juice taken as fruit would require perhaps an hour of chewing, and therefore an hour of tasting and smelling. Unless you drink it very slowly and carefully, all but a fraction of the tasting is lost. The same goes even more for vegetable juices. The body has difficulty dealing with the sudden massive influx of highly absorbable fruit sugar. I recommend taking fruit juice either highly diluted, or in slow sips that are carefully "chewed."

Milk is more a food than a drink, and a sacred one at that. It contains a lot of nourishment and should not be drunk merely to relieve thirst. With its complex and evocative flavor, milk is an especially instructive food on which to practice the Yoga of Eating. Note that conventional pasteurized, homogenized cows' milk comes with severe health and ethical concerns. If you ever have a chance, use attentive tasting to compare it to whole raw milk from pastured cows. Some authorities argue that many of the common allergies to dairy products are related to the highly processed state of conventional milk, which is made even more problematic by the way we consume it. Children often gulp it down ice-cold and, because we parents insist it must be good for them, in large quantities. This is the opposite of how it should be. For one thing, milk is meant to be drunk warm, and in small sips, never gulped—thing of a nursing baby! Large quantities are fine for some people, but this should come from the body's desire, not a rule of "four a day." Finally, I believe that fresh, unsoured milk has a vibration unsuitable to many adults. On a biochemical level this may manifest as decreased lactase production (sour milk, yogurt, kefir, buttermilk, and cheese have less lactose, so lactase isn't needed), but even for a lactose-tolerant adult like me, there is something odd about fresh milk. Sometimes I go through phases where it is repugnant to me, where it seems too raw for the adult body. In any case, milk is a special food that adults should consume consciously, not habitually.

Soy milk, **rice milk**, and the like are increasing in popularity, despite serious concerns among dissident nutritionists about their health effects. Both contain mineral blockers and enzyme inhibitors that make them difficult to digest, while soy also contains estrogen-mimicking chemicals that may disrupt endocrine function. These concerns are beyond the scope of this book, however. In any event, soy milk and rice milk are highly concentrated foods that, like fruit juice, should be drunk in tiny sips and small quantities. Also like fresh fruit juice, the homemade product seems to have a different quality than the store-bought version.

The Yoga of Eating precludes any hard-and-fast rules prohibiting any given food; however, if I had to issue a blanket recommendation against any single food item, it would be **soda pop**. Again, the details of its health hazards are beyond the scope of this book; I'll just opine that it is probably the single most damaging item on the American menu. An illuminating exercise is to drink some soda with full attention and sensing. For me it is hard to drink more than a couple sips before it begins to taste awful. Ironically, modern soda pop is made in imitation of traditional beverages—root beers and ginger ales—that were fermented from natural sugars and herbs. These were very healthful beverages, not necessarily alcoholic, loaded with enzymes, vitamins, beneficial microorganisms, and electrolytes.

Beer, particularly unfiltered homebrew, is a generally healthful drink in moderate quantities. Like other fermented foods and drinks, it can actually be an aid to digestion. However, virtually all modern beer uses a fairly potent medicinal herb, hops, which is a sedative and sexual depressive not suited to some constitutions. Traditionally, there were dozens of herbs commonly used in beer, all with different tonic, flavoring, healing, or even psychotropic properties. The appreciation and exploration of the ways of fermentation is both an art and a yoga.

Wine is another potentially healthful beverage for its vitamins, antioxidants, and digestive stimulation. Again, home-fermented wine is probably the best, since most commercial wines have sulfite and pesticide residues. The subtle nuances of flavor in wine, and the culture of appreciation that has grown up around it, also makes wine a gateway into the yogic sensing and appreciation of food.

One way to practice sensing the subtle effects of food on the body is through the use of **herbal teas**. These can delicately modulate one's state of body and mind. The variance in potency between packaged commercial herbal teas and ones you make from herbs you gather yourself can be astonishing—further evidence that its entire history of production, and not just its taxonomic classification, affects the symphony of vibrations embodied in a food.

As the adverse health effects of **caffeine** and **alcohol** are well known, it is understandable that most diet books recommend against them. But to evaluate these substances on a more inclusive level, it is necessary to consider their social, religious, and medicinal roles in a given culture. I discuss this in some depth in the appendix "The Illness Seeks the Medicine." A full discussion of the overt consciousness-altering effects of alcohol, caffeine, and other psychotropic chemicals within a yogic framework is beyond the scope of this book.

For now I will just observe that caffeine in **coffee** and theobromine in **tea**, said to affect the body identically, actually have fairly significant differences that one can easily notice with the application of a little yogic attention. I don't know whether there is any scientific basis for this observation. Both have, among other effects, the ability to aid concentration. When does one need help in concentrating? For one, when you are doing something you really aren't interested in. When a baby is absorbed in a fascinating task such as pulling off her sock, she doesn't need coffee to maintain total concentration. But if you are poring over lists of figures in an office cubicle, your mind naturally wants to escape and coffee can help you stay focused. One might even argue that the modern office could hardly run at all without coffee.[6] For some people, this means that quitting coffee has implications beyond health and diet. A caffeine high can accompany a sense of well-being, that things are okay after all, that one need not do anything right now about disturbing issues that had seemed urgent minutes before. An otherwise intolerable existence becomes tolerable without removing any of the underlying conditions. Fortunately, or unfortunately, caffeine is not powerful enough to maintain this effect for long.

The use of tea goes back thousands of years in eastern Asia, and has accumulated a corpus of ritual and aesthetics probably exceeding French wine culture in the fineness of its development. Depending on one's individual psycho-physical makeup, the negative effects of tea's theobromine may be far outweighed on the physical level by its potent antioxidant content, and on the aesthetic level by its infinitely delicate nuances of flavor and aroma. The appreciation of fine tea is a tao and a yoga unto itself.

In spite of all the information I have presented above, remember that whatever the beverage, the only authority is your own body. Enjoy exploring the flavors and effects of the whole range of beverages, but since truly healthful beverages are not easily available, don't be surprised if you end up drinking mostly water.

Unfortunately, the story does not end there, because these days it is especially important to carefully taste and evaluate your water. In most of the world today, the quality of tap water and even of bottled water is severely compromised. There is much evidence that common additives such as chlorine and fluorides are poisonous, not to mention the pharmaceutical residues, fertilizer residues, heavy metals, toxic wastes, and other contaminants often found in our water supplies. On the other hand, distilled water is a highly processed substance that may actually leach minerals from your body. (It might be temporarily appropriate for a cleansing phase, however.) The information out there on water filtration systems is confusing and often contradictory, and mineral water sources are not necessarily pristine. The senses of smell and taste, plus the deeper intuitional senses underlying them, are therefore essential allies in finding the optimum source of this life-giving liquid. Even supposedly odorless substances affect the vibrational quality of water, so see what your body can tell you about the water you drink.

Chapter 18

Supplements

Those who break off a piece of nature lay hold of something that is dead, and, unaware that what they are examining is no longer what they think it to be, claim to understand nature.
— Masanobu Fukuoka

Most books on eating and nutrition devote copious space to the subject of vitamins, minerals, and other nutrients. They promote the idea that foods are good for you because of the vitamins or other substances they contain: spinach is good for you because it has beta carotene and iron, kelp because it has iodine and zinc, flax seeds because they have omega-3 fatty acids, sprouts because they have lots of enzymes, and so on.

If it is the vitamins or other food elements that are healthful, then why not just eat them in pure form? That's the idea behind most nutritional supplements: we can extract or synthesize the nutritional essence of foods to remedy deficiencies in our diet or achieve super health. From this perspective, there is little reason to eat whole, organic, unprocessed foods, because you can get your vitamins (and whatever other substances you need) from a pill or in "fortified" food products. For example, most white flour has minerals and B vitamins added to it to replace those lost with the wheat germ in processing. Breakfast cereals are laced with up to one hundred percent of the recommended daily allowance of a multi-

117

tude of vitamins and minerals. Outside the mainstream, the same thinking prevails. According to various dietary philosophies, if only we had more enzymes, or chlorophyll, or anti-oxidants, or water-soluble fiber, or any of hundreds of other substances trumpeted in the latest books on diet, perfect health would be ours.

Yet, when people take multivitamin supplements, pills, powders, herbal extracts, or whatever, they don't ordinarily experience dramatic, lasting improvements in their health. Even if you take pills with every known vitamin and mineral, your chances of living to a hundred or avoiding cancer improve only marginally, if at all. You certainly don't become Superman. When people start to take responsibility for their health they often start with supplements, but invariably they move on to something else. Clearly there is something wrong with the vitamin theory of health.

That the physiological effects of food correspond in a predictable way to certain of their more basic constituents is an idea fully consistent with the reductionistic paradigm that still dominates medical science today. Under this paradigm, the primary explanation is the reductionistic one. For example, recent research has shown cruciferous vegetables, particularly broccoli, to have anti-cancer properties. The question "Why?" is answered by analyzing various molecules found in broccoli to find which might disrupt cancer cell growth. Why does broccoli fight cancer? Because it contains sulforaphane. The next step is to isolate or synthesize sulforaphane, because then you can get the cancer-fighting power of twenty heads of broccoli packed into one pill. With pills like these, who needs broccoli?

Of course, research scientists won't stop their search with sulforaphane, but will continue looking for other anti-cancer components of broccoli to more fully explain its effects. There is another possibility, however, one that is outside the dominant paradigm of medical research. What if the *whole plant* has protective effects against cancer that exceed the effects of any subset of its components? Perhaps all the chemical constituents of broccoli, everything that makes broccoli *broccoli*, act synergistically to protect the body in a unique way. Constituent A might interfere with cancer cells' growth mechanism, constituent B might prevent side effects of constituent A from harming normal cells, constituent C might provide enzymatic resources needed for constituent A to take effect, and so on.

Sometimes, of course, a given vitamin can dramatically improve a health condition: vitamin C for scurvy, vitamin B_1 for beriberi, niacin for pellagra, vitamin D for rickets, vitamin B_{12} for pernicious anemia, etc. In fact, vitamins were mostly discovered via diseases of deficiency. That makes them unique in having direct, dramatic, identifiable effects on health. What of other substances whose deficiency effects are more general, more subtle? Foods contain thousands, even millions, of distinct organic molecules that interact in very complex ways. Remove some of them from this enormous interdependent web, and its overall function begins to deteriorate.

Vitamins are among the millions of molecules in food. In whole foods, they never exist in isolation, but rather together with various synergens. Vitamin C always accompanies bioflavonoids, rutin, and tyrosinase, among other substances. We now "officially" define vitamin C as ascorbic acid, but actually ascorbic acid is just part of a complex group of interacting molecules that compose the real vitamin C. Interestingly, pure ascorbic acid often won't even cure scurvy![1] Vitamin E defined as tocopherols is another example—it is merely the antioxidant protector of a group of molecules accompanying a selenium atom.

Think of it this way: the few dozen vitamins recognized today represent a tiny fraction of the thousands of vitamins the human body requires. Taking just the known vitamins, without the thousands of others found in whole foods, generates biochemical imbalances in the body. Worse yet, purified, fractionated vitamin components like ascorbic acid taken over the long term could draw down the body's reserves of their natural synergens without which they cannot fully function.

From the perspective of the Yoga of Eating, no knowledge of chemistry is necessary to reject the use of super-concentrated food supplements or vitamins, except as medicines for temporary remedial use (if then). The reason is simple: it is impossible to fully taste and experience them as foods. The body does not know what it is getting.

Wheat grass juice is a popular super-food that you can buy in tablet form. Without even tasting it, you can swallow an amount of wheat grass essence equivalent to perhaps half an hour of chewing actual grass. The chewing and tasting is what allows the body to adjust to and absorb this powerful food. Experiencing the wheat grass with the senses vibrationally aligns the body and the food.

Supplement pills, powders, and liquids are usually designed to eliminate any strong taste. For example, you can get cod liver oil or wheat germ oil in gel capsules so you don't have to taste it. They even make deodorized garlic tablets. These products deprive your body of the information it needs to use them, and preempt any feelings—disgust or pleasure—through which your body could tell you whether the supplement is helpful or not.

We as a society are enamored of supplements because we hope we can enjoy good health without making any changes in diet or lifestyle. The idea is to pop a few pills, and keep shoveling down the junk food with impunity. Such thinking ignores the organic interdependence among all body systems, and among physical, mental, emotional, and spiritual health.

It is the height of arrogance to suppose that we know better than the body what it really needs. Taking supplements amounts to forcing quantities of potent substances literally down our own throats, bypassing the normal safeguards against imbalance and overconsumption. If you eat too much of a certain substance from a natural food source, that food will become repulsive to you. It will taste disgusting. In other words, you will get sick of it. But since one pill tastes like another—that is, like nothing at all—nothing stops you from continuing to take it. You are groping in the dark.

Sometimes it is necessary to take powerful, concentrated foods to heal the body. Given today's impoverished soils and environmental pollution, such foods might even be a necessity for even the healthiest eaters. In general, though, eating powerful foods should be a rather intense experience, for the taste will be concentrated as well. These substances will be unpalatable unless that's what your body really hungers for.

It is no wonder then that Chinese herbs sipped in the traditional way as infusions of whole herbs are generally recognized as far more potent than the exact same doses gulped down in powdered form. Any product missing its taste is suspect. Taste is not an afterthought, not incidental to the effects of foods or herbs, but rather an inseparable part of their essence.

Chapter 19

Processing

That on which commerce seizes is always the very coarsest part of a fruit—the mere bark and rind, in fact, for her hands are very clumsy.[1]

— Henry David Thoreau

Many dietary philosophies inveigh against food processing, whereby natural whole foods are changed into denatured, devitalized, partial foods. Food processing takes food away from its natural state, and introduces substances that were never meant to be part of the human diet. From the point of view of the Yoga of Eating, processing can also alter or mask the original flavors of food, distorting the body's perceptions of it. Since cooking is a form of processing, some authorities go so far as to advocate a raw food diet, which was the diet of our pre-human ancestors and is still the diet of our closest biological relatives, the great apes.

Food processing goes far beyond what happens in the factories of the food industry. Transporting a food, for example, is a kind of processing. Genetic manipulation, even traditional selective breeding, is a form of processing—pre-processing, you could call it. Also in this category we can include any soil preparation, fertilization, weeding, or tending; even pruning a tree. And after the food reaches our kitchens, we cut, juice, cook, or otherwise process it. According to this strict definition, almost all food that we eat is processed to some degree, the sole exception being

123

wild foods picked in their natural habitat. Most vegetables and fruits are actually highly processed even when fresh-picked, by the careful breeding of generations of farmers. They are very different from their wild relatives. Strictly speaking, the only time most of us eat a truly unprocessed food is when we pick wild blackberries or eat dandelion greens from the yard.[2]

It is true that industrial processing compromises much of the energy in food. White flour and white rice are less nutritious than their whole-grain counterparts. Even the gentle processing we call cooking depletes food of enzymes and water-soluble vitamins.[3] Wild foods such as dandelion often have many times more vitamins and minerals than cultivated foods such as spinach. Given these facts, some advocate a diet consisting wholly of raw, unprocessed foods. Other diets, for example the "Paleolithic diet," attempt to emulate the eating habits of our hunter-gatherer ancestors living in a state of nature. The thinking is that we would be much healthier if we ate the foods we were "meant" to eat, the foods that millions of years of evolution have designed us for. No other animal eats cooked food—why should the human physiology be any different?

Upon deeper examination this logic breaks down. Let us return to the concept of the "symphony of vibrations." What kind of lifestyle, what state of being, does a raw foods diet or Paleolithic diet nurture? With what symphony of vibrations does it harmonize?

Fire and the Human Condition

The earliest form of food processing was cooking, and to cook food you need fire. There is considerable scientific controversy over the earliest use of fire, with estimates ranging from 1.5 million years ago to 300,000 years ago. Whatever the earliest use, it is fairly certain that by 125,000-150,000 years ago the use of fire for cooking was widespread.[4] Interestingly, this is also the approximate date of the appearance of the first anatomically modern humans.[5] (The other human species, the Neanderthal, appeared 200,000 years ago, also well after the first established use of fire.)

124

It is therefore safe to say that human beings have *always* cooked their food.

What is it to be human, anyway? Recent discoveries confirm that we are not the only animal to use tools, but we are surely the only animal to use fire. Fire was the precursor to the exponential rise of technology from the Neolithic onward; its use is the hallmark of civilization. In the most primitive setting, the light of the campfire defined a zone of security, the human zone, a circle of domesticity; outside of it was the wild. With the mastery of fire, human beings ceased to be wild. We ceased to be animals. And since the earliest use of fire was for cooking, we should not be surprised to discover that cooked foods nourish a state of being that is also domestic and civilized, distinct from raw animality.

Cooking has been around so long that there has been ample time for human anatomy and physiology to genetically adapt to cooked foods. Indeed, it may very well be that the adoption of fire and other technology precipitated the speciation event that changed *Homo erectus* into *Homo sapiens*. It is possible that we are adapted to eating cooked food; it may be written into our very biology..

A completely unprocessed diet—that is, a diet consisting of wild foods in the natural raw state—is compatible with a state of being that is as well raw and wild. It is the state of being our primitive ancestors enjoyed, before the long coevolution between *Homo sapiens* and technology. To go back to a *Homo erectus* diet without also adopting the rest of a *Homo erectus* lifestyle introduces disharmony. Now I think it is a perfectly fine thing to revert to a primitive life. If you wish to give up such trappings of civilization as clothes, heating, books, shoes, hot water, and so forth, then a totally unprocessed diet might be perfect.[6] But if you plan to hold onto even some of the technologies of fire (basically everything but stone tools), then you probably will also need a diet to which fire is applied—a diet including cooked foods.[7]

You cannot expect to shift to a diet of raw, wild foods and live a modern lifestyle. It is impossible, in fact: if you really wanted to gather your own food, you'd have to give up a normal career and living routine. Today we live anything but a raw, wild lifestyle.

Processed Food, Processed Lives

The goal of the Yoga of Eating is not to eliminate all processed food from our lives. Rather, it is to find the degree of processing consistent with the life we live, and the life we want to live. To nourish a modern lifestyle, some processing of food is necessary. Different activities require different foods and different kinds of processing. Cooked grains, for example, were wholly absent from the human diet until perhaps 12,000 years ago, but some authorities claim they are wonderful for nourishing sustained mental work of a kind unnecessary for pre-civilized peoples.[8] Thus, cultivation of grain—the hallmark of civilization—is also necessary, perhaps, to support a civilized state of being for the individual. It makes beautiful sense.

Cooked, domesticated foods represent a very gentle degree of processing. Unfortunately, most of us consume foods that are far, far more highly processed. The extreme processing represented by today's highly refined packaged foods—subjected to intense chemical processing and very high heat, adulterated with synthetic additives, shipped across continents and oceans—fosters a state of being that few would call healthy. Many of the degenerative diseases that afflict modern humans are traceable to our diet of highly processed food, but the impact goes much deeper than that. Remember the principle of karma: What are we saying yes to by eating a highly processed diet?

A diet of over-processed food goes hand in hand with living an over-processed life. In modern society, all of us live, to some degree, a processed life; that is, a life in which social, economic, and political forces channel our intrinsic spontaneity. Even in ancient tribal societies, this was true to some extent. But today many people's lives are so highly processed that they have completely lost touch with their life purpose. Just think, what is the main reason people have increasingly turned to prepared foods—frozen dinners, restaurant takeout, and fast food? Convenience. Here is a handy definition of convenience: other people doing things for you. A convenience store: other people have pre-chosen a limited range of products for you and shipped them to a nearby location—

moved them for you. Convenience foods: other people have prepared them for you. Convenience comes down to other people bringing things to you and doing things for you. Things we once did ourselves we now pay others to do for us. We even pay people to care for our children. Why? Because it is more efficient, because we just cannot afford to spend the time. We are too busy. Our time is increasingly channeled, funneled into a narrow set of activities: work, commuting, and so forth. Mandatory activities dominate, while our range of optional activities, our range of freedom, gets narrower and narrower, more and more superficial. Freedom devolves into meaningless choices between Wal-Mart or K-Mart, brand A or brand B, NBC or CBS; the "freedom" to drive to work in a Toyota or a Ford. Meanwhile, we are no longer sovereign over meaningful areas of life, not even our thoughts and opinions—yes, we think processed thoughts and hold processed views, simplified for our convenience. This is what I mean by living a processed life.

Whether applied to life or to food, mass processing makes bland what was once varied, unique, and unpredictable. To spice them up, we add to our mass-produced lives the delusional excitement of sports fandom, Santa Claus, shopping sprees, designer fashions, celebrity news, trips to Disney World, TV dramas, new cars, new computers, and new furniture. And to our mass-produced food, we add flavors and sensations that are equally devoid of substance: concentrated sweeteners, MSG, and the myriad chemical additives produced by the flavor industry. In remarkable parallel to our overstimulated lives, these additives offer a superficial zest and intensity not backed by substance. The nutrition, the pith, the stuff of life is gone. Just as TV commercials lie when they associate hipness and happiness with, say, a brand of clothing, so also do the exciting flavor (and color) additives of processed food lie to the body, promising vast constellations of nutrients and compounds that are not there. In a natural food, flavors are markers, inseparable from its entire chemistry, by which the body understands that food. The ethyl-2-methyl butyrate in an apple, for instance, is not incidental to the fruit, but an integral product of the whole biochemistry of that species.[9] Taken in isolation, as the flavoring in a

127

packaged food, the ethyl-2-methyl butyrate promises the body an apple, but no apple is to be found. After a lifetime of such letdowns, the body learns to distrust food flavors and loses the ability to distinguish healthful foods by taste and smell. Fortunately, we can recover this ability by avoiding MSG and artificial flavors, and refocusing on the fuller, more complex flavors of natural foods.[10]

To complete the analogy with the rest of life, we feel a comparable letdown when images of success, excitement, and happiness do not jibe with the reality. The eventual response is cynicism, a sense that nothing is real and that nothing really matters. In parallel with my advice on food, we can only recover a sense of authenticity by avoiding life's phony flavor enhancers and coming back to the fundamentals of nature, family, solitude, friends, play, and creative work.

The Anonymous Power of Money

Processed food and processed lives are connected to a persistent expansion of the role of money in society. Centuries ago in the West, and more recently in the Third World, significant functions of household economy took place outside the realm of money. The vast majority of people grew most of their own food, made most of their own clothes, built their own houses, created their own entertainment, and most certainly cooked their own meals, cleaned their own houses, and cared for their own children. What people could not do for themselves was covered by community and kin. One by one, these functions have become monetized (that is, given over to professionals) to the point where even the intimate functions of cooking, cleaning, and child care are often performed by paid outsiders.[11] The domain of our lives over which we are sovereign continues to shrink.

Money is an anonymous energy. Whereas earlier forms of exchange—barter and social reciprocity—depended on personal relationships and community ties, money, by definition, is a universal medium of exchange. We still depend on other people to survive, but because our relationships with them are mediated primarily by money, those people are interchangeable. It does not matter who works at the grocery store, who drives the delivery truck to the store, who operates the machinery at the canning plant, or who grows the food. You don't need to have a personal relationship with these people, because you *pay* them to do it. Therefore, full participation in today's money economy leads quite naturally to feelings of loneliness and isolation. More than ever before in history, *you* are interchangeable too. Someone else can be paid to do what you do.

If you don't want your goals, your dreams, your relationships, and your very life to be so highly processed, consider a shift in your diet away from industrial mass-processing, and toward home-processing. If you believe as I do that a strong web of close personal relationships is fundamental to human happiness, then you would be wise to affirm such relationships in your diet. Replace the standardized cooking of fast food restaurants with home cooking. Replace industrial food preservation with home fermentation, pickling, and canning. Replace California-grown or Mexico-grown produce with garden vegetables. Eat food grown and processed by yourself, your family, your friends, or people in your community. Your body can be your ally in this shift, because once you mentally move away from a standardized, anonymous, processed life, then the corresponding convenience foods won't taste as good anymore.

You cannot change one thing without changing everything. As soon as you begin to practice the Yoga of Eating, you find that you want to prepare your own food. Convenience foods are no longer palatable. But you cannot abandon processed foods without also abandoning, step by step, a processed life. Food can be a fulcrum about which your entire life changes. Eat whole, natural, organic, home-processed foods and many social functions will become awkward. You'll gravitate towards gatherings where people share your food preferences. Cook more, and you'll need to spend more time in the kitchen, more time in the home. You will need to become less busy. You will need to exert your autonomy to reclaim genuine choices in your life.

The causality works the other way too. If you have no desire to live a less processed life, then you will find it basically impossible to sustain a diet of home-cooked foods either. The mechanism for this result is not so mysterious. You just won't have the time. When you rush from one commitment to the next, fast food on the go is a natural choice, perhaps a necessary choice.

We moderns live fractured lives. The minute division of labor, in which even basic functions of food preparation, housekeeping, and child care have become the commoditized province of specialists, separates us from ourselves. We are losing sovereignty over more and more personal aspects of our lives. Strangers produce nearly everything we eat and everything we use. We are disconnected from the source of our food and our things. To reintegrate our fractured lives, our fractured selves, our fractured communities, and our fractured souls is indeed a deep and important yoga. For yoga means union, and the Yoga of Eating extends beyond bodily integrity to encompass every aspect of our individual and collective lives.

Chapter 20

The Yoga of Cooking

Good men are released from their sins when they eat food of-fered in worship; but the wicked devour their own evil when they cook for themselves alone.
— Bhagavad Gita

If a woman could see the sparks of light going forth from her fingertips when she is cooking and the substance of light that goes into the food she handles, she would be amazed to see how much of herself she charges into the meals that she prepares for her family and friends.
— Maha Chohan

Cooking is the most ancient way of processing food. The food processing industry evolved in large part to replace home cooking with industrial mass-cooking. To make mashed potatoes from scratch, we must clean, perhaps peel, slice, cook, and mash them with other ingredients. A box of instant mashed potatoes embodies most of these steps already—all that's left for the cook to do is add hot water.

On a vibrational level we are closely linked to family members. Our

131

symphonies of vibrations share many common chords. Any time or energy put into food imbues it with the vibrations of the people and machines doing the work. Food prepared by loved ones therefore harmonizes better with one's own vibrations than food prepared by strangers. This is something we can taste. No matter how well it is prepared, restaurant food just tastes different. It tastes like restaurant food. Home cooking tastes like home. And mother's cooking has its own specialness. When we eat home cooking we are ingesting love, devotion and caring. Of course, the cook might be angry that day, or under pressure, or resentful, but the vibrations imbued go beyond surface emotions to include the intimacy of family. In a way, it is obscene to eat food prepared by anonymous strangers.

The soul needs the nourishment of the loving vibrations generated by home cooking. Of course it is okay to eat sometimes with friends—indeed, sharing food together is perhaps the most ancient bond of friendship, and nourishing in its own way—and even, occasionally, at a restaurant. But to eat strangers' food day in and day out depletes the spirit and eventually, the body. It is connected to feelings of alienation, of being lost in a crowd, of meaninglessness, of a cold, impersonal world. The greater the anonymity, the worse the depletion: a small neighborhood restaurant where everyone knows you personally, where the cook cares about you and cares about the food, is far superior to a national franchise outlet. Again, consider: What are you saying yes to?

Remember that money is the great anonymizer. It is what allows relationships to be anonymous.

Just as food is the greatest expression of Nature's generosity, cooking and serving food to others is a primal act of human nurture. At a deep biological level, sharing food equates to love.

Because it is an expression of love, preparing food for others is a sacred act. Our culture has denigrated cooking for centuries, first belittling it as "women's work" and then, later, as a trivial inconvenience to be avoided as much as possible through technology. But actually, cooking is not a lowly, but a high, venerable, and sacred activity.

When you cook for loved ones, what kind of universe are you saying yes to? One where people are cared for without expectation of repayment—a fundamentally generous universe. When you cook for others, not for money, not contriving to garner gratitude, not for any selfish advantage, but simply to nourish them on a physical level, you are generating very strong positive karma.

Unfortunately, because our society so demeans cooking, it is hard to approach it without some resentment, without some feeling that your time could be better spent, that you are above this. To make a yoga out of cooking, first realize that this mundane activity is very spiritual, not something to get out of the way, but to approach with sincerity and devotion. Express your caring by using the most nutritious ingredients according to your current understanding. Do not demand you be appreciated, but let your satisfaction be in the pleasure of others.

In the yoga tradition this is known as karma yoga, the yoga of selfless service, the most powerful of all yogic paths. That cooking is so devalued, and cooks so taken for granted, makes this yoga all the more profound. Moreover, you can easily practice this yoga every day, in the midst of family life, and its master yogis are all around us among the grandmothers of the world.

Chapter 21

Food is Only Food

With coarse rice to eat, with water to drink, and my bended arm for a pillow: I have still joy in the midst of these things.
— The Analects of Confucius

There are people who strictly deprive themselves of each and every eatable, drinkable, and smokable which has in any way acquired a shady reputation. They pay this price for health. And health is all they get for it. How strange it is. It is like paying out your whole fortune for a cow that has gone dry.
— Mark Twain

Thou shouldst eat to live; not live to eat.
— Socrates

Throughout this book I have described food as a repository of karma, as a primeval means of comfort and connection, and as something that nourishes who we are and who we wish to be in the world. Have I thus turned eating into a weighty responsibility, something deadly serious?

The Yoga of Eating does not seek to elevate food to a position of primary importance in life. Socrates' adage that we should "eat to live, not live to eat" contains much wisdom. Food is just one of the ways we nourish ourselves, define ourselves, and interact with the world. To all these aspects of our living and being, we should apply the same mindfulness, the same trust, and the same joyful acceptance of universal providence that I have advocated in the realm of food. Yes, eating is a sacred act, but no more so than anything else if you hold as I do that the world— creation—is itself sacred. And by sacred I just mean that it is to be treated as if it mattered. Can you imagine how full and rich life would be, if we only believed that it mattered?

So please, do not turn reverence for food into an obsession that diminishes the sacredness of any other part of life.

Chances are, the deepest solution to your problems is not to be found in your diet. Yet to the extent that each aspect of life is a microcosm of the whole, it is likely that many of your problems will indeed have a dietary dimension. Dietary changes often coincide with major life changes in general. Many people stop snacking and overeating when they find a calling or a life partner, or when they leave a bad job or a bad relationship. But if the fundamental problem is a bad relationship, changing your diet probably isn't going to help. In such a situation, overindulging on sweets (for example) might be a symptom of the relationship problem; it might be an indicator of what is missing. And it will only end when we remove the underlying conditions from which it arises.

The quest for health and the perfect diet can easily become an obsession. If our lives harbor a major problem that is too scary to face, we might turn to an area that is less intimidating. For many people, diet is an area that seems much more under their control, much less complicated to face, than painful family problems. In the extreme case of anorexia, control over the body's appetites compensates for a perceived lack of control in the rest of life. It is like the Sufi tale of Mullah Nasrudin, searching for his key under the streetlight instead of in the shadows where he lost it. Rarely do we find the courage to venture into the shadows, even if it leaves us searching forever in places where the answers cannot be found.

We often find the same phenomenon when it comes to dealing with problems on a social level. Whereas nutrition barely merits even a single course in many medical schools, many health crusaders go to the opposite extreme in blaming poor diet for nearly every physical, mental, and social ill. Depression, violence, and attention deficit disorder have all been attributed to various dietary factors. Meanwhile, activists in other areas attribute the same social ills to excessive television viewing, or to modern birthing practices, or to our system of schooling. It is time to recognize that all these causes are just as equally effects. They are all part of a pattern, a gestalt. Diet is not incidental to the rest of life. For a child separated from his mother in the maternity ward nursery, raised by childcare workers, babysat by the television set, and subjected to an authoritarian school system, a junk food diet is almost inevitable. It fits right in. A nutrition activist might say, "What good is school reform when the children's diets make them incapable of paying attention?" An educational reformer might say, "What good will better diets do when there's nothing worth paying attention to?" Enlightened reformers in all areas recognize the interdependency of all our social maladies, and build alliances rather than dismissing other activists' work as less important.

The Russian-Armenian mystic G.I. Gurdjieff was once quoted as saying, "To change one thing, everything must be changed." A more positive corollary of this proverb is, "Change one thing, and everything else *will* change." Change any one of the ruling junta of birth, television, diet, and schooling, and change will call out to the others as well. An excellent diet is simply not compatible with sickness in any other part of life.

So where does this leave the unfortunate woman who binges and snacks to avoid facing difficult life issues? Can she, by changing her diet, automatically change everything else? Not quite. To the extent that her junk food habit made her abusive relationship and unsatisfying job bearable, quitting that habit will make these problems even more painful! The new discrepancy between her diet and her way of life will generate a powerful tension. But if she doesn't make the now-more-obvious changes in her work and relationship, neither the tension nor the pain will diminish. Eventually, the willpower by which she maintains her diet will fail, and she will gratefully succumb to the analgesic effect of her former eating habits.

If on the other hand she faces and resolves the real problem in her life, a cascade of positive changes will follow. The whole pattern of her life shifts once she divorces that abusive husband, or gathers the courage to say yes to a new vocational opportunity. In situations like these, it is not uncommon for health complaints to clear up as if by magic, for pounds of fat to melt away, and for the diet to change spontaneously in response to new circumstances. In the absence of other changes, the Yoga of Eating simply brings into sharper relief the deeper problems in our lives. So in one sense, the Yoga of Eating is inconsequential—it doesn't solve the real problems. Come on, you and I know that eating really isn't all that important. In fact it is almost nothing. Yet in another sense, the Yoga of Eating can be a key to everything, because there is no aspect of our lives that does not cast a shadow onto our diet.

The same applies to physical health. Health is important primarily insofar as we are able to achieve our life's purpose, to live the life we ought to live. Beyond that, of what use is it? Someday we all die anyway, and a lifetime of good health is little consolation for a lifetime of missed opportunity. We are embodied, I believe, for a reason. It is when poor health interferes with the fulfillment of our reason for being that recovering health must become a top priority.

It is futile to seek out physical health and dietary perfection as a surrogate for self-fulfillment. At best diet & health are but part of this path, and indeed there are times when the health, safety, and even survival of the body must be sacrificed for more important things. Health and proper food must sometimes yield to a more encompassing integrity.

Chapter 22

Health and the Quest for Wholeness

In ancient times, those who wished to illuminate the world with virtue first brought order to their nations. Wishing to order well their nations, they first harmonized their families. Wishing to harmonize their families, they first cultivated themselves. Wishing to cultivate themselves, they first rectified their minds. Those who wished to rectify their minds first made their intentions sincere.
— Confucius

In an age rent by grave environmental and social problems, conscientious people understandably look askance at "health nuts" concerned with perfecting their bodies even as the world is falling apart around them. Obsession with physical health, they reason, is a vain and foolish luxury: vain for its elevation of a superficial aspect of one's self; foolish because, after all, good health can't protect a person from environmental disaster, social unrest or, eventually, old age and death. Better to devote oneself to the world's pressing problems and not be so selfish.

On the other hand, spiritual practitioners and health enthusiasts look at social activists and wonder, "How can they pretend to be saving the world when they cannot even heal themselves?" Would you trust a doctor who were himself sick? Indeed, there is something hypocritical about an environmental activist, say, who is vindictive, small-minded, and domi-

139

neering in her personal relationships, or the social crusader who is a neglectful husband and distant father.

Earlier in *The Yoga of Eating* I wrote: ". . . if body and soul are not separate, then to heal the body at the deepest level is a work of the soul, and to listen to and learn from the body is to become closer to one's Self." This implies that the health nut's quest is not so straightforward, not so simple as discovering the secret of correct diet, or the true secret tradition of Qigong, or some special super-food, or any other amendment to life as usual. We soon discover that to fully heal ourselves even on the grossest physical level, it becomes necessary to bring all aspects of life into greater integrity and wholeness.

Etymologically speaking, the word health means nothing other than "a state of wholeness." Any conception of health that depends on separating a person's physical, mental, emotional, familial, social, and spiritual being, cannot truly be health in the deepest sense. Physical health, for example, is impossible if you harbor burning resentments. It is impossible to be completely healthy when your relationships are not healthy. It is impossible to have completely healthy relationships when the society in which they are embedded is sick. Nor can our society be healed without also healing its relationship to the earth. Therefore, even the most physically oriented practice, if sincere, inexorably extends into every corner of life: relationships, means of livelihood, diet, social interaction, and political activity.

The reverse is also true: no genuine healing of society or the planet is possible without a concomitant transformation on the individual level. Even if the planetary environment were miraculously restored, in the absence of a spiritual transformation we would just go about ruining it again. Our poisoned world is a reflection of our poisonous thoughts and feelings. You can't build a solid house on a rotten foundation, and our minds are the foundation of our common world. Yes, we must address the crisis of the earth, but at the same time we must also address the source of that crisis in ourselves.

The same goes for social change: if, say, a utopian socialist state were imposed without eliminating the roots of greed and competitiveness in each one of us, the old injustices would quickly reappear. In fact, one could argue that all such attempts have failed precisely because a social revolution cannot revolutionize the deepest reaches of the human heart; that the urge to power, to domination, to profit can only be cleansed from the inside out.

This is not to discourage a person whose practice or activism is limited to just one realm, be it the meditation cushion, the dinner table, or the arena of social activism. I do not demand that you scurry to extend yoga—the quest for wholeness—into all realms of individual and collective life. Demanding is unnecessary because the yoga grows on its own. It reveals contradictions that your life may have harbored for decades; and it makes these contradictions intolerable. This illumination is an inevitable product of any branch of sincere yogic practice.

For example, social, environmental, or political activism is a form of karma yoga, the yoga of selfless service to others. Its most evident focus is to bring fragmentation into unity on the transpersonal level. The focus cannot be limited to that, however, because one's ignorance and prejudice cripple efforts to do good or to help others. How will you know whether you are actually serving others, or just gratifying a selfish desire? You know only to the extent that you are honest to yourself, that you know your own mind. Therefore, karma yoga eventually demands some kind of inner practice.

The same is true of the Yoga of Eating. Food has a political dimension that manifests when you try to seek out sources of healthful food. A major premise of this book is that the bad karma embodied in food tastes bad, too. Listening to my body has compelled me to change my venues of social interaction, to become active in developing and sharing sources of natural whole foods, and to work to change unjust laws governing food production. It is simply impossible for me to eat the way I wish to without getting involved in these larger issues.

When a person decides to learn from and trust the body, it may be that no belief system is left intact. For example, if your body tells you certain foods are toxic, and a little reading about such things as hydrogenated oils confirms this feeling, then you are left to wonder why food corporations promote these substances, why the medical profession doesn't warn us about them, and why the government permits them. Our faith in the integrity of these institutions is shaken, and along with it, perhaps our faith in the rightness of our vocation, education, modes of social interaction, and everything else embedded in this society. Of course, you can ignore the contradictions between, say, changing to a more natural diet and your job at a soda manufacturer, but if your practice of the Yoga of Eating, or indeed of any yoga, is sincere, these contradictions will become harder and harder to deny.

Work on ourselves inextricably involves work on our physical and social environment, including career and art, marriage and friendships, and relationship with parents, society, and the earth. One might even say that the world has been given us as an instrument for accomplishing inner work. Remember, matter is not separate from spirit, nor soul from flesh. Our lives in the world are significant, spiritually significant. The world has been given to us as a vehicle of worship, and every act counts. Our actions are prayers, prayers far more substantive than any we say kneeling by our beds, and they cannot fail to have an effect.

Chapter 23

Relaxing Into Change

The new moon like a knife
Carries the old moon on his arm.
I was young.
   — Basho

In the beginner's mind there are many possibilities; in the
expert's mind there are few.
   — D.T. Suzuki

Dislodging a green nut from a shell is almost impossible, but let
it dry and the lightest tap will do it.
   — Ramakrishna

The Indian philosopher Krishnamurti said that change imposed upon oneself is not true change, because it comes from where one is right now. Authentic change requires not willpower and forcing, but surrender, acceptance, trust, and courage. It requires the willingness and courage to let change happen. It is a step into the unknown, a trusting of something beyond ourselves. There is no guarantee.

In the Yoga of Eating we trust the body to guide dietary change. It is a step into the unknown because you don't know where it will take you,

143

or what beliefs you will have to drop about what is healthy or right. It is also a trusting of something greater than yourself—your body, which is far vaster than your conscious mind. We wonder doubtfully, "If I let my body have its way, will it lead me astray?" In a society where the media tells you your body is ugly and the medical establishment tells you your body is unreliable, it is especially hard to trust your natural appetites.

I have argued in this book that your body naturally seeks what is best for it. Furthermore, your body will tell you what it wants (if you'll only listen). Your body is wise. Let alone, without the imposition of some concept of what it should or shouldn't be, your body will move towards its natural state of beauty and wholeness.

Not just the body but all natural things, when left undisturbed, move naturally toward beauty and wholeness. If you don't keep repaving it every few years, an ugly parking lot will crack, grass will come up, and after 100 years or so you'll probably have a beautiful forest. Your body is the same way. Stop "paving it over" with artificial ways of being, stop trying to be other than what you are, and it will move towards its natural state of health and beauty. It happens sooner than you think. Why else is rest so healing? Have you ever noticed how beautiful a sleeping person looks?

The body's self-healing ability is truly amazing. If your car has a flat tire or a leaking crankcase, you can't let it rest in the garage for a few days and expect it to get better. But the body can repair itself—if you let it, if you can let go of the knots responsible for the illness. My faith in the body's capacity for self-repair runs contrary to many social and medical assumptions. Our medicine regards the body as a source of trouble, something that must be constantly monitored, adjusted, and fixed. Thus we have come to accept as normal an old age defined by decrepitude and decline.

Such an old age is only normal because modern life rarely leaves the body undisturbed. We constantly disturb, disrupt, and impose upon our bodies. We go around with chronic tensions and holdings which, over time, congeal into disease. We impose destructive dietary habits on our bodies in disregard of our natural appetites. Instead of letting our true selves shine through, we habitually wear facial expressions and adopt postures and mannerisms to show a contrived image of ourselves to the world. These habitual facial expressions congeal into the lines of old age. And on our minds we impose attitudes and belief systems that corral our thoughts into the same old ruts, crippling our ability to learn.

Deep relaxation reverses these habits. In the body, this means searching for tension, knots, and holdings, attitudes and postures, and letting them go, bringing the body as close as possible to its natural, undisturbed state. When we do this, we liberate the body's self-healing power, as its natural energies, now unrestrained, flow to where they are needed the most. In relaxation, the body begins to reestablish balance.

In the mind, relaxation means letting go of habitual thought patterns, anxieties, and systems of belief, including the customary avoidance of uncomfortable thoughts ("I won't think about that! I won't go there!") as well as the chronic clinging to interpretive beliefs about the world, which filter the facts according to preconceived notions of truth. By letting go of these holdings and relaxing the mind; that is, by identifying less strongly with our beliefs, we open the mind to new thoughts, new ideas, and new understanding, reversing the otherwise inevitable progression of mental ossification.

The Yoga of Eating is itself a kind of a relaxation encompassing both physical and mental elements. Not manipulating, controlling, imposing upon, or dismissing the body's messages, it trusts the body to move towards its natural rest state: beauty and wholeness. Everything you need to know about eating is already there inside of you.

Thus the fundamental method and practice of the Yoga of Eating is to listen to your body-soul, trusting the tools of taste, smell, and intuition, not imposing any specific expectations, not expecting any specific results. The results will come of themselves. Meanwhile, enjoy the delights so freely available in the form of food, a gift that never ends.

Appendix I

The Illness Seeks the Medicine

From looking at your neighbor and realizing his true signifi-
cance, and that he will die, pity and compassion will arise in you for
him and finally you will love him.
— G.I. Gurdjieff

Where lowland is, that's where water goes. All medicine wants
is pain to cure.
— Jelaluddin Rumi

Can true humility and compassion exist in our words and eyes
unless we know we too are capable of any act?
— St. Francis of Assisi

As individuals and as a society we seem drawn to behaviors that
contribute to our own destruction, behaviors that keep us in a low, unhealthy, depressed state of existence. Seeing the destruction wrought by
diets, habits, and lifestyles, we decide to make a change. A kind of self-
disgust motivates this effort: disgust at our moral failings, our weak willpower, our selfish indulgence.

One person might be disgusted at his frequent outbursts of rage, in
which he shouts at his loved ones and speaks venomous words causing

permanent harm in his relationships. "What's wrong with me?" he thinks. Another person might feel disgust at her smoking addiction, which makes her feel filthy and weak-willed. Another woman is disgusted at her inability to stand up for herself in economic and personal relationships. "Something is wrong with me," she says, "Why do I let people take advantage of me?"

And of course, disgust for ourselves implies disgust for other people, for who's perfect? Self-judgment implies a high standard for everyone, not just oneself. Sometimes judgmentality is covert, part of a disingenuous ploy of false modesty. Other times it is quite overt. We denounce reckless drivers, speeding through quiet residential neighborhoods, as if they were some kind of monster, their behavior incomprehensible. We look with contemptuous self-satisfaction at the obese woman loading her supermarket cart with potato chips. We cluck at the wanton self-disrespect of so-and-so's promiscuous sister, and shake our heads in censorious disapproval at the latest statistics for marital infidelity.

In judging others there is a sense of self-affirmation, a self-image built from "I would never do that." In that statement is coded a profound lack of unconditional self-acceptance, and the secret dread that, Yes, I would in fact do that, or even the shameful knowledge: I have done that before.

Please do not read into these words a contempt for judgmental people. That would be hypocritical! Yet the reason not to judge, measure, despise, and envy others is not to avoid being hypocritical; it is not because you "shouldn't," it is not because it's "wrong"—all of these reasons, too, are freighted with self-judgment and judgment of others.

Let me restate: Do not tell yourself that you shouldn't be judgmental. You'll tie yourself up in knots, because when you really dig down into what "shouldn't" means you will very likely discover an implicit judgment of judgmental people.

Moreover, in the end it is not only futile, but also unnecessary to enforce a policy of non-judgmentality upon yourself. That's because judgmentality withers away of its own accord when compassion arises, and compassion arises, naturally and effortlessly, from the sober, unsentimental understanding of the origin of a person's behavior.

Such understanding may be encapsulated into two aphorisms, which I beg you not to dismiss lightly, as they are subtle and many-layered:

(1) You would do as others do, if you were they.

(2) The illness seeks the medicine.

Most people object to the first statement immediately. "No," they protest, "if I were Andrea Yates I would have sought professional help, I wouldn't have drowned my five children in the bathtub."[1] In making this statement, we import our own experience of being human into the role of Andrea Yates. What it means is, "If Andrea Yates were I, she would not have done that." But Andrea Yates was Andrea Yates, and how can you possibly know what it was like to be her? It is almost beyond imagining, but I have tried very very hard to imagine it. I have tried to imagine the depths of a despair so utterly relentless, a cosmic hopelessness so all-consuming, a despondency so abject, complete, and merciless, that I could drown, one by one, the very children whom I'd comforted and loved, fed and changed, taught and protected day after day, year after year, watching their personalities unfold; those familiar faces, dependent on me, their imperfect caretaker. And I imagine the act itself: averting my eyes from their puzzlement, giving way to fear, then terror, and then blank death; closing my ears to the others crying as they wait their turn, not understanding, knowing only that something is very, very wrong, yet still clinging, perhaps, to a piteous trust. And then, after the crime, an agony of remorse too enormous to face and too acute to avoid, a hell without hope. I have tried very hard to imagine this, because that is my yoga. What would a person have to feel, how would a person have to be, to commit such an act? Who can say what history of her soul brought her to such a state? How can you possibly know that you—not as you but as Andrea Yates, complete in the entire context of her existence—would not have done as she did? As for myself, I do *not* know.

I have chosen for my example perhaps the most horrifying crime imaginable. It is much easier to imagine circumstances in which I'd speed through a quiet residential neighborhood. I imagine feeling that there's never enough time, and perhaps a sense of invulnerability, and self-importance—taking charge in a world where I feel stripped of power.

It is easy to imagine being obese and loading up my shopping cart with potato chips and candy. Perhaps needing a comfort food in a world of too little comfort; having a sweet treat to compensate for a lack of sweetness in life, for hopes gone sour and relationships turned bitter. Being good to myself, in the only way I know how (maybe that's how my parents showed love) in a world that is rarely good to me.

It is easy to imagine being promiscuous in a world bereft of intimacy, seeking a union of souls in a society that tears us apart; and, finding only the tiniest hint of such a union in the physical union of uncommitted sex, seeking it again and again; trying to assuage the loneliness; wanting to feel loved, wanting to love another unconditionally as in the first blush of infatuation. There are many scenarios I can imagine in which promiscuity would come naturally.

When you put yourself fully in another's place, imagine what it is like to be them, and feel what they feel, there is no possibility of judgmentality. Others will sense that, and trust you, and be amazed that you know things about them they have never told you. Herein also lies humility, a sincere humility arising simply from an understanding of the fact: "I would surely do as you do, if I were you."

It is accurate enough for the present purpose to say that all of us are damaged souls. To a greater or lesser degree, we have suffered the hurts of the world. The response to this hurting, which we might judge as a flaw, sin, or crime; despicable, contemptible, or disgusting; is, as the above examples illustrate, a natural reaction, perfectly understandable. And not only understandable, but wise even, and touching. Thus we come to the second aphorism, "The illness seeks its medicine."

Let us start with drug abuse. Typically, our society regards alcohol and drug addiction as either a morally deplorable weakness or as a "disease," a term which, in this day and age, strongly implies helpless victimhood. Yet there is another way to view drug use that is neither arrogant nor patronizing, and is, as I shall argue, in the end far more empowering: Drug use is a form of self-medication, and drug addiction is essentially similar to dependency on any medicine that keeps one functioning "normally."

It is curious and highly significant that the same word, "drugs," should apply both to pharmaceutical medicines and to substances of abuse such as alcohol, cocaine, heroin, etc. Even in conventional medicine, the active constituents of such things as opium and cocaine, or their chemical analogs, have important medical applications. Consider the possibility that drugs such as alcohol are indeed powerful medicines with far broader applicability than ordinarily admitted.

In medicine, heroin's chemical brother morphine and its cousin codeine are used a painkillers. Considering pain in a broad sense, is it any wonder that tortured souls are drawn to these drugs?

Very many alcoholics and addicts I have known are extraordinary people, of exceptional intelligence and sensitivity and, very often, exceptional musical or artistic talent. How can we denser folk blame them for seeking to deaden their sensitivity to a very painful world?

Alcohol too deadens pain, but its effects are not limited to just that. Alcohol can also help open us up, relax our boundaries, let down our guard. I know many people whose sole moments of intimacy, outside of sex, occur under the influence of alcohol. Many people are able to speak certain truths (for better or for worse) only when drunk. Moreover, alcohol can open us up another way too, to poetic inspiration. Ancient and tribal cultures universally considered alcohol to be a divine gift, a "spirit" (and this is indeed the origin of the word "spirits" to refer to liquor).

Lest the reader think I am advocating drug use, let me hasten to add that under ordinary circumstances, drugs and alcohol address the symptoms only. Narcotizing pain does nothing to address its source. Many pharmaceutical medicines also just treat the symptoms of disease, and even those that treat a proximate cause, say penicillin for ear infections, may not address the deeper cause. (Why is this person susceptible to ear infections?) Most medicines, especially for chronic conditions (and that is what I'm talking about here), merely alleviate the symptoms; they make the condition more bearable. For a time, they allow people to function "normally."

People with drug dependencies probably have a much better reason for self-medication than most of us imagine. Instinctively, they are drawn to the substance that addresses the symptoms of their damaged souls. When I see an addict, very often I see a child just trying to make it stop hurting.

We may now take a conceptual leap beyond chemical substances, to consider as medicines other kinds of addiction, distraction, indulgence, stimulation, and lifestyle.

Once driving through New York on a major six-lane highway at midnight, I witnessed one motorcycle after another zoom by at close to a hundred miles an hour through the heavy traffic, weaving among the cars plodding at a mere 65 mph—a form of recreation few people would approve of, I'm sure. To me, though, there was something beautiful and poignant about these young thrill-seekers risking life and limb for fun. Get past the judgmental attitude of "There's just something wrong with them," and "I would never do that." Think instead, How would life have to be, for me to do that? Think, What kind of spiritual malady would that address the symptoms of? Imagine a life hopelessly bland and unpromising, a dull and pointless education, dead-end job prospects; a spirit broken, almost, by controlling institutions, and exploding out to reclaim itself. When we condemn youthful rebelliousness, or dismiss it with a knowing, patronizing wink, we deny that rebellion can be right and just. Perhaps their rebellion, destructive as it is, shows that against all odds there is life in them yet; perhaps we can see in these motorcycle daredevils the heroism and indomitability of the human spirit, contorted almost beyond recognition. Why does this behavior attract them and not me? Is it just that I'm more blessed with some elemental virtue called responsibility? Or does it address a particular lacking or wrongness in their experience of the world? Perhaps they are medicating themselves, as best they know how.

So ready we are to condemn human weakness! Elsewhere I have

written about the pernicious narcotizing and soul-stealing effects of television. Yet we can understand television too as a medicine: a palliative to a bleak and barren social landscape, an imitation hearth to assuage the piercing loneliness of life in modern society.

In *The Yoga of Eating* I discuss the allure of that dietary poison, excessive refined sugar. A pale imitation, is sugar, of the sublime sweetness of intimacy and spiritual connection; but when relationships are sour and life is spiritually bland (as it is so often in materialistic culture), the yearning for even imitation sweetness is overpowering.

Consider now the minor vice of constantly looking at yourself in the mirror. Think about it—what illness would that ease? How would you have to be, to check yourself out in every reflective surface that goes by? A reflection provides reassurance: Yes, I am here. Yes, I am okay. I look fine. I can like myself. True, it is a paltry reassurance in the face of the yawning pit of self-alienation that afflicts us all, to some extent, but for a moment at least it eases the anxiety.

To say that these medicines are palliatives, and engender deepening dependency without true healing, is only a partial truth. Partial, but illuminating nonetheless. Obviously, riding a motorcycle through traffic at a hundred miles an hour does not resolve the underlying discontent and ennui, which themselves result from complex, deep-seated social, karmic, and biographical factors. Eating candy does nothing to bring spiritual sweetness into life, nor does eating "treats" alleviate an underlying feeling of undeservingness. Television, while momentarily making you feel less lonely, will not enrich your social life—on the contrary, it separates you even more from other people, at the very least in the sense that watching TV is usually a solo activity. Fantasy role-playing games and escapist novels cannot take you away from a dull or painful reality forever. In the same way that narcotic drugs deaden pain without affecting its source, all of these activities alleviate the symptoms of the illness (at least temporarily), thus making the illness itself easier to bear.

None of these medicines work forever. Eventually, a given medicine or class of medicine becomes either toxic, or ineffectual due to buildup of resistance, or unusable due to a change of circumstances. For example, sweets become toxic with the onset of type II diabetes. Build-up of resistance to television (and other diversions) manifests as boredom. Mirrors become unusable (for the purpose described above) if someone suddenly notices he has aged, or suffers a disfiguring accident that renders him ugly (in his own eyes). In one way or another, the medicine fails. Then the underlying issues rise to the surface.

Sooner or later a crisis will strike. It is inevitable. That is why the medicines I speak of are not quite mere palliatives, but steps on the path of genuine healing. Each represents a necessary stage for a given individual. And the crisis they eventually lead to is a true medicine, one that brings the deep wounds to the surface for healing. Very often a clue to the deep wounds is present in the earlier, palliative medicine; its failure illuminates just what was missing, just how a person was not whole. Before the medicine fails, even the symptoms of our soul wounds are obscure to us, not to mention the wounds themselves. In the failure of the medicine, the quality of the pain finally emerges. Ahh, one thinks, all along I was just lonely. All along I was angry. All along I was afraid. The behaviors that society sees as flaws and that I see as palliative medicine all of a sudden make sense.

When you begin to see through a medicine in this way (thanks to a crisis or imminent crisis), then, and only then, is it time to give it up. If you try to remove the medicine before you are ready to face the wound, before you can handle the pain unmedicated, then the inevitable result is an intensification in the suffering, which drives you back to the medicine or to a new, substitute medicine. That is why forceful intervention to keep an alcoholic sober is rarely successful. Next time you start to nag someone to quit her addiction or other vice, ask yourself whether you want to deprive a sick person of her medicine. (Never take away someone's medicine unless you see very clearly that it no longer serves them.)

Rather than take away someone's medicine, instead remove the conditions that make the medicine necessary. In the case of friends, and particularly relatives and intimate partners, you yourself might be contributing to those conditions. For example, by keeping secrets and telling lies, we exacerbate the loneliness and hunger for intimacy of those in our lives. Another way to help someone is to illuminate the wound underneath the behavior, the quality of the pain. When you see a self-medication not working for someone anymore, you do them a favor by pointing that out, making its uselessness more obvious.

As for your personal vices, unless and until you have seen through them to the quality of the pain underneath, do not coerce yourself into quitting them just because you "should," because they might be just what the doctor ordered. Consider that the soul is wise, and has sought out the right medicine for its condition. Be kind to yourself, and never practice self-deprivation for its own sake.

On the other hand, when the medicine does fail, do not shy away from what truths the failure reveals. When the medicine stops working, stop using it. When the time comes, do not be afraid to *be with the pain.* The truth cannot harm you, but the truth can hurt! It is okay to hurt. Ah, the bitter truth! Do you, dear reader, harbor some bitter truth, too terrible to admit right now even to yourself? The devices you use to keep it out of sight and out of mind are your medicine. Someday they won't work anymore. The truth will out.

The failure of a medicine is often dramatic: a serious illness, a close brush with death, the humiliating discovery of an affair, a mental breakdown, a destructive fit of violent rage, financial bankruptcy. Sometimes, as in the case of Andrea Yates, it seems intentional. Other times people subconsciously engineer a disaster: a businessman, long neglectful of his family, blinds himself to the fact that a deal is doomed, inviting his own bankruptcy. Even when the occurrence appears completely arbitrary—an airplane crash, for instance—perhaps the soul has sought out that situation too.[2]

If the medicines of thrill-seeking, alcohol, sweets, television, mirrors, and so forth—habits, peccadilloes, and indulgences—can be likened to long-term palliative medication, then the dramatic blunders and catastrophes of life are like major surgery. Their consequences, such as remorse, physical pain, grief, and imprisonment make it impossible to forget the presence of a wound. Suffering of this sort is a true medicine, not because it heals, but because it leaves us no choice but to heal.

At this point, we might replace the adage "The illness seeks its medicine" with another: "The illness *is* the medicine." Or rather, the *symptoms* are the medicine. Separation from God is painful. It is painful not to be whole. This pain, which we can avoid or muffle only temporarily, inexorably compels us to try again and again to heal ourselves. We try as best we know how, learning along the way, discarding measures that we discover to be useless, digging deeper and deeper toward the source of the pain.

Compassion for others and, even more, for oneself, doesn't require overlooking flaws or ignoring the shadow side. Innate divinity does not lie apart from our most shameful sins; it lies within them. Underneath everything you are and everything you do is a sweet, innocent being, doing its best to cope with the confusing world into which it has wandered. You are a pure, earnest child plunged into a maelstrom with only the most exiguous of threads connecting you back to your Mother. Do not judge yourself too harshly, for you have done your best with the knowledge available to you.

When you can understand every action, of yourself and others, as the touchingly naive response of an innocent baby-in-an-adult-body to a world gone incomprehensibly wrong; seeking, as all creatures will, to avoid pain in a very painful world; buffeted, like milkweed in a storm, by environmental forces vastly dwarfing the power of any single individual; concealing a fathomless well of loss and private sadness; taking on a measure of difficulty and suffering at the very edge of one's capacity; and yet, heroically, striving, surviving, and transcending circumstances beyond any reasonable expectation; then you will see glory in every person, a divine and radiant beauty; and you will realize that like all people, you do even as God would do, if God were you.

Appendix II

The Ethics of Eating Meat: A Radical View

Just now
A rock took fright
When it saw me.
It escaped
By playing dead.
   — Norbert Mayer

Most vegetarians I know are not primarily motivated by nutrition. Although they argue strenuously for the health benefits of a vegetarian diet, many see good health as a reward for the purity and virtue of a vegetarian diet, or as an added bonus. In my experience, a far more potent motivator among people ranging from idealistic college students, to social and environmental activists, to adherents of Eastern spiritual traditions like Buddhism and Yoga, is the moral or ethical case for vegetarianism. Enunciated with great authority by such spiritual luminaries as Mahatma Gandhi and by environmental crusaders such as Frances Moore Lappé, the moral case against eating meat seems at first glance to be overpowering. As a meat eater who cares deeply about living in harmony with the environment, and as an honest person trying to eliminate hypocrisy in the way I live, I feel compelled to take these arguments seriously.

A typical argument goes like this: In order to feed modern society's enormous appetite for meat, animals endure unimaginable suffering in conditions of extreme filth, crowding, and confinement. Chickens are packed twenty to a cage, hogs are kept in concrete stalls so narrow they can never turn around. The cruelty is appalling, but no less so than the environmental effects. Meat animals are fed anywhere from five to fifteen pounds of plant protein for each pound of meat netted—an unconscionable practice in a world where many go hungry. Whereas 1/6 acre of land can feed a vegetarian for a year, over three acres are required to provide the grain to raise a year's worth of meat for the average meat-eater. Sometimes, those acres consist of clear-cut rain forests. The toll on water resources is equally grim: the meat industry accounts for half of US water consumption—2500 gallons per pound of beef, as compared to 25 gallons per pound of wheat. Polluting fossil fuels are another major input into meat production. As for the output, 1.6 million tons of livestock manure pollutes drinking water—and let's not forget the residues of antibiotics and synthetic hormones that are increasingly showing up in municipal water supplies. Even without considering the question of taking life (I'll get to that later), the above facts alone make it clear that it is immoral to aid and abet this system by eating meat.

I will not contest any of the above statistics, except that they only describe the meat industry as it exists today. They constitute a compelling argument, not against meat-eating, but against the *meat industry*. For in fact there are other ways of raising animals for food, ways that make livestock an environmental asset rather than a liability and in which animals do not lead lives of suffering. Consider, for example, a traditional mixed farm combining a variety of crops, pasture land, and orchards. Here, manure is not a pollutant or a waste product; it is a valuable resource contributing to soil fertility. Instead of taking grain away from the starving millions, pastured animals actually generate food calories from land unsuited to tillage. When animals are used to do work—pulling plows, eating bugs, and turning compost—they reduce fossil fuel consumption and the temptation to use pesticides. Nor do animals living outdoors require a huge input of water for sanitation.

In a farm that is not just a production facility but an ecology, livestock has a vital role to play. The cycles, connections, and relationships among crops, trees, insects, manure, birds, soil, water and people on a living farm form an intricate web, *organic* in its original sense, a thing of beauty not easily lumped into the same category as a 5000-animal concrete hog factory. Any natural environment is home to animals *and* plants, and it seems reasonable that an agriculture that seeks to be as close as possible to nature would incorporate both. Indeed, on a purely horticultural farm, wild animals can be a big problem, and artificial measures are required to keep them out. Nice rows of lettuce and carrots are an irresistible buffet for rabbits, woodchucks, and deer, which can decimate whole fields overnight. Vegetable farmers must rely on electric fences, sprays, traps and—more than most people realize—guns and poison to protect their crops. Even if the farmer refrains from killing, raising vegetables at a profitable yield requires holding the land in a highly artificial state, cordoned off from nature.

Yes, one might argue, but the idyllic farms of yesteryear are insufficient to meet the huge demand of our meat-addicted society. Even if you eat only organically raised meat, you are not being ethical unless your consumption level is consistent with all of Earth's six billion people sharing your diet.

Such an argument rests on the unwarranted assumption that our current meat industry seeks to maximize production. Actually it seeks to maximize profit, which means maximizing not "production" but "productivity"—units per dollar. In dollar terms it is more efficient to have a thousand cows in a high-density feedlot, eating corn monocultured on a chemically-dependent five-thousand-acre farm, than it is to have forty cows grazing on each of twenty-five two-hundred-acre family farms. It is more efficient in dollar terms, and probably more efficient in terms of human labor as well. Fewer farmers are needed, and in a society that belittles farming that is considered a good thing. But in terms of beef per acre (or per unit of water, fossil fuel, or other natural capital) it is not more efficient.

In an ideal world, meat would be just as plentiful perhaps, but it would be much more expensive. That is as it should be. Traditional societies understood that meat is a special food; they revered it as one of nature's highest gifts. To the extent that our society translates high value into high price, meat should be expensive. The prevailing prices for meat (and other food) are extraordinarily low relative to total consumer spending, both by historical standards and in comparison to other countries. Ridiculously cheap food impoverishes farmers, demeans food itself, and makes less "efficient" modes of production uneconomical. If food, and meat in particular, were more expensive then perhaps we wouldn't waste so much—another factor to consider in evaluating whether current meat consumption is sustainable.

So far I have addressed issues of cruel conditions and environmental sustainability, important moral motivations for vegetarianism to be sure. But vegetarianism existed before the days of factory farming, and it was inspired by a simple, primal conviction that killing is wrong. It is just plain wrong to take another animal's life unnecessarily, it is bloody, brutal, and barbaric.

Of course, plants are alive too, and most vegetarian diets involve the killing of plants. (The exception is the fruit-only "fruitarian" diet.) Most people don't accept that killing an animal is the same as killing a plant though, and few would argue that animals are not a more highly organized form of life, with greater sentience and greater capacity for suffering. Compassion extends more readily to animals that cry out in fear and pain, though personally, I do feel sorry for garden weeds as I pull them out by the roots. Nonetheless, the argument "plants are alive too" is unlikely to satisfy the moral impulse behind vegetarianism.

It should also be noted that mechanized vegetable farming involves massive killing of soil organisms, insects, rodents, and birds. Again, this does not address the central vegetarian motivation, because this killing is incidental and can in principle be minimized. The soil itself, the earth itself may, for all we know, be a sentient being, and surely an agricultural system, even if plant-based, that kills soil, kills rivers, and kills the land is as

160

morally reprehensible as any meat-oriented system, but again this does not address the essential issue of intent: Isn't it wrong to kill a sentient being unnecessarily?

We might also question whether this killing is truly unnecessary. Although the nutritional establishment looks favorably on vegetarianism, a significant minority of researchers vigorously dispute its health claims. An evaluation of this debate is beyond the scope of this article, but after many years of dedicated self-experimentation, I am convinced that meat has been quite "necessary" for me to enjoy health, strength, and energy in most phases of my life. Does my good health outweigh another being's right to life? This question leads us back to the central issue of killing. It is time to drop all unstated assumptions and meet this issue head-on.

Let's start with a very naïve and provocative question: "What, exactly, is wrong about killing?" And for that matter, "What is so bad about dying?"

It is impossible to fully address the moral implications of eating meat without thinking about the significance of life and death. Otherwise we are in danger of hypocrisy, stemming from our separation from the reality of death behind each piece of meat we eat. The physical and social distance from slaughterhouse to dinner table insulates us from the fear and pain the animals feel as they are led to the slaughter, and turns a dead animal into just a piece of meat. Such distance is a luxury our ancestors did not have: in ancient hunting and farming societies, killing was up close and personal, and it was impossible to ignore the fact that this was recently a living, breathing animal.

Our insulation from the fact of death extends far beyond the food industry. Accumulating worldly treasures—wealth, status, beauty, expertise, reputation—we ignore the truth that they are impermanent and therefore, in the end, worthless. "You can't take it with you," the saying goes, yet the American system, fixated on worldly acquisition, depends on the pretense that we can, and that these things have real value. Often only a close brush with death helps people realize what's really important. The reality of death reveals as arrant folly the goals and values of conventional modern life, both collective and individual.

It is no wonder, then, that our society, unprecedented in its wealth, has also developed a fear of death equally unprecedented in history. Both on a personal and institutional level, prolonging and securing life has become more important than how that life is lived. This is most obvious in our medical system, of course, in which death is considered the ultimate "negative outcome," to which even prolonged agony is preferable. I see the same kind of thinking in Penn State students, who choose to suffer the prolonged agony of studying subjects they hate, in order to get a job they don't really love, in order to have financial "security." They are afraid to live right, afraid to claim their birthright, which is to do joyful and exciting work. The same fear underlies our society's lunatic obsession with safety. The whole American program now is to insulate ourselves as much as possible from death—to achieve security. It comes down to the ego trying to make permanent what can never be permanent.

Digging deeper, the root of this fear, I think, lies in our culture's dualistic separation of body and soul, matter and spirit, man and nature. The scientific legacy of Newton and Descartes holds that we are finite, separate beings; that life and its events are accidental; that the workings of life and the universe may be wholly explained in terms of objective laws applied to inanimate, elemental parts; and therefore, that meaning is a delusion and God a projection of our wishful thinking. If materiality is all there is, and if life is without real purpose, then of course death is the ultimate calamity.

Curiously, the religious legacy of Newton and Descartes is not all that different. When religion abdicated the explanation of "how the world works"—cosmology—to physics, it retreated to the realm of the nonworldly. Spirit became the opposite of matter, something elevated and separate. It did not matter too much what you did in the world of matter, it was unimportant, so long as your (immaterial) "soul" were saved. Under a dualistic view of spirituality, living right as a being of flesh and blood, in the world of matter, becomes less important. Human life becomes a temporary excursion, an inconsequential distraction from the eternal life of the spirit.

Other cultures, more ancient and wiser cultures, did not see it like this. They believed in a sacred world, of matter infused with spirit. Animism, we call it, the belief that all things are possessed of a soul. Even this definition betrays our dualistic presumptions. Perhaps a better definition would be that all things *are* soul. If all things are soul, then life in the flesh, in the material world, is sacred. These cultures also believed in fate, the futility of trying to live past our time. To live rightly in the time allotted is then a matter of paramount importance, and life a sacred journey.

When death itself, rather than a life wrongly lived, is the ultimate calamity, it is easy to see why an ethical person would choose vegetarianism. To deprive a creature of life is the ultimate crime, especially in the context of a society that values safety over fun and security over the inherent risk of creativity. When meaning is a delusion, then ego—the self's internal representation of itself in relation to not-self—is all there is. Death is never right, part of a larger harmony, a larger purpose, a divine tapestry, because there is no divine tapestry. The universe is impersonal, mechanical, and soulless.

Fortunately, the science of Newton and Descartes is now obsolete. Its pillars of reductionism and objectivity are crumbling under the weight of 20th century discoveries in quantum mechanics, thermodynamics, and non-linear systems, in which order arises out of chaos, simplicity out of complexity, and beauty out of nowhere and everywhere; in which all things are connected; and in which there is something about the whole that cannot be fully understood in terms of its parts. Be warned: my views would not be accepted by most professional scientists, but I think there is much in modern science pointing to an ensouled world, in which consciousness, order, and cosmic purpose are written into the fabric of reality.

In an animistic and holistic world view, the moral question to ask ourselves about food is not "Was there killing?" but rather, "Is this food taken in rightness and harmony?" The cow is a soul, yes, and so is the land, and the ecosystem, and the planet. Did that cow lead the life a cow ought to lead? Is the way it was raised beautiful, or ugly (at least, according to my current understanding)? Allying intuition and factual knowledge, I ask whether eating this food contributes to that tiny shred of the divine tapestry that I can see.

There is a time to live and a time to die. That is the way of nature. If you think about it, prolonged suffering is rare in nature. Our meat industry profits from the prolonged suffering of animals, people and the Earth, but that is not the only way. When a cow lives the life a cow ought to live, when its life and death are consistent with a beautiful world, then for me there is no ethical dilemma in killing that cow for food. Of course there is pain and fear when the cow is taken to the slaughter (and when the robin pulls up the worm, and when the bear downs the caribou, and when the hand uproots the weed), and that makes me sad. There is much to be sad about in life, but underneath the sadness is a joy and a fullness of being that is dependent not on avoiding pain and maximizing pleasure, but on living rightly and well.

It would indeed be hypocritical of me to apply this to a cow and not to myself. To live with integrity as a killer of animals and plants, it is necessary for me in my own life to live rightly and well, even and especially when such decisions seem to jeopardize my comfort, security, and rational self-interest; even if, someday, to live rightly is to risk death. Not just for animals, but for me too, there is a time to live and a time to die. What is good enough for any living creature is good enough for me. Eating meat need not be an act of arrogant species-ism, but consistent with a humble submission to the tides of life and death.

If this sounds radical or unattainable, consider that all those calculations of what is "in my interest" and what will benefit me and what I can "afford" grow tiresome. When we live rightly, decision by decision, the heart sings even when the rational mind disagrees and the ego protests. Besides, human wisdom is limited. Despite our machinations, we are ultimately unsuccessful at avoiding pain, loss, and death. For animals, plants, and humans alike, there is more to life than not dying.

Endnotes

Chapter 2 - Body and Soul

1. Quoted by Michael Shermer in *Scientific American*, February 2002, p. 35.

2. This interpretation is borrowed in large part from Daniel Quinn's book, *Ishmael*.

3. And that is why freedom of religion has come to mean so little. If matter and spirit, body and soul are separate, then who cares what your "spiritual" beliefs are? They are inconsequential to the world. Apply them to life and you will soon find just how little freedom of religion there is. For example, try citing freedom of religion in going naked in public, altering your consciousness with psychotropic plants, letting your lawn revert to its natural state, or walking God's Good Earth in violation of "property rights." As long as religion only concerns the disembodied "soul" it poses little threat to anyone.

4. This is not to imply that seriously ill people are less "spiritually healthy" than the rest of us. An apparently healthy person might simply not be ready for the illness to manifest. Some traditions speak of an "energy body," a template for the physical body in which imbalances eventually manifest as physical symptoms, perhaps years or even lifetimes in the future. Therefore, for all we know, a sick person may be closer, and not further, from wholeness than an apparently healthy person.

Chapter 3 - Birth and Nurturance

1. For a deeper journey into the psychodynamics of birth, I highly recommend the works of Stanislav Grof, in particular *Realms of the Unconscious*.

Chapter 4 - Food and Personality

1. No killing of the tree, that is. The living cells of the fruit itself are of course still dying.

2. This is the conventional ranking, though personally I believe that the soil, which is disturbed or even murdered in conventional chemical horticulture, is a highly conscious being.

3. To maintain a herd of dairy cows, something must be done with all the males. Beef production is therefore almost always a byproduct of milk production.

4. These reports will seem fantastical to the skeptical reader. Anyone who assumes "It isn't true because it couldn't be true" is unlikely to seriously examine the evidence, which is not easily dismissed when taken at face value. However, the truth or falsity of such stories has little relevance to the thesis of this book.

5. http://www.beyondveg.com/billings-t/bio/billings-t-bio-1a.shtml.

6. Referenced in the skeptic website "The Apologetics Index": http://www.gospelcom.net/apologeticsindex/b12.html. For fun, in the same sitting try reading a skeptical source on Breatharianism followed by the writings of an exponent of Breatharianism such as Jasmuheen's *Living on Light*.

Chapter 5 - The Karma of Eating

1. Belief in reincarnation is not necessary for a correct understanding of karma. What is necessary is a concept of the self that is greater than the linear, biographical person most of us conceive ourselves to be. Really what karma comes down to is that all your acts *matter*. That is a tremendously liberating belief; as the Sufis say, "When you realize God sees everything, you are free."

Chapter 6 - The Natural Breath

1. The breath, in fact, could be viewed as another kind of eating, in which we take in a substance necessary for life and expel waste products for the environment to recycle.

2. "Qigong" literally means "work with qi" while pranayama means "prana control." It is highly significant that both words, "qi" and "prana," can refer not only to breath but to a kind of spiritual energy that is believed to interpenetrate all living creatures, and indeed the entire universe. Other languages also imply this identity between breath and spirit or energy; in English, for example, the word "respiration" means literally to "refill with spirit."

Chapter 7 - The Central Practice

1. The constant hurrying and, you could say, existential unease I speak of is not an accidental byproduct of busy modern life, but its central defining feature. Even if there is a lull in the schedule, the mind races onward, constantly interrupting itself with one anxious demand after another, trying to tie up all the loose ends and make sure everything is okay.

2. Joseph Chilton Pearce connects this to the way we commonly discipline toddlers. When a toddler learns a mechanical task, she concentrates one hundred percent of her awareness on it. Unfortunately, whatever the toddler is learning might be annoying or inconvenient to the parent, or downright dangerous. Very often the toddler is interrupted with a scolding: "Get your hands away from that socket now!" Eventually she associates concentration with a scolding or worse, and learns it is best not to concentrate so fully. The entrainment function is attenuated. Sometime go to a playground where there are parents with their toddlers, and listen to the incessant chorus of "No!"

3. One wonders whether palate desensitization might also occur with heavily spiced traditional cuisines. I suspect the effect is less than one might guess. For example, in much of Sichuan the food is incredibly hot: often stir-fried hot peppers don't just garnish a dish—they *are* the dish! Toddlers may be given water red with the infusion of hot peppers. To a person accustomed to such foods, however, the hotness is not dominant. The pain receptors on the tongue become desensitized, but the taste buds are unaffected, as is the

olfactory apparatus. Other highly seasoned cuisines affect primarily the sense of smell, not taste, whereas modern junk food stimulates mainly tongue receptors for sweetness, saltiness, and *gan* or *umami*, a fifth taste recognized only recent in the West as a "meaty" taste that is also stimulated by monosodium glutamate.

4. Many fascinating examples of plant communication are given by Stephen Harrod Buhner in his marvelous book, *The Lost Language of Plants*.

Chapter 8 - Making It Practical

1. Here I am advocating "the path of surrender." What about the element of discipline that exists in all spiritual traditions? The two paths intertwine, and ultimately may be understood as one. A full discussion of this would occupy a very long essay, but if you'd like a hint, just consider how difficult it is to fully relax. It is simple but it is not easy. In fact, try it right now. Relax your jaw muscles and keep them relaxed. Now relax your thumbs. And now think of what time you plan to get up tomorrow, and your first obligation of the day. Do you have it firmly in mind? Good. Now, is your jaw still relaxed? Didn't think so.

Chapter 10 - Distinguishing Appetites from Cravings

1. Moshe Feldenkrais, founder of the Feldenkrais Method, makes a similar point in his discussion of "cross-motivation." I quote: "Many people eat themselves to death trying to relieve the tension due to the longing for approval or recognition, or the anxiety due to insecurity. They do not eat to relieve the tension of hunger." *The Potent Self*, p. 27.

2. Sometimes you might find that the craving seems to be coming from somewhere outside of the body entirely, almost as though it were an external force, a demon. What a far cry from the common assumption that the body betrays us by craving unhealthy foods.

3. But it can't be a trick. The permission must be real, not to be conditional upon moderation. I once read the following teaching story, I cannot remember where: "Rabbi, you told me I would become famous if I turned my back on fame. This I have done, yet I am still not famous. Why?" The rabbi

responded, "You have turned your back, but you are still looking over your shoulder!"

4. Actually the promise "This was the last time" is worse than just a distraction. Because the promise is never kept, the addict feels hopelessly weak-willed and his unconscious mind grows increasingly disconnected from the ego.

Chapter 11 - Loving the Body, Loving the Self

1. The mania for purity and "super-health" is especially prominent among various raw food cults. Others have written extensively about the psychology and physiology of raw food-ism (see for example www.beyondveg.com). Perhaps the best medicine for a person inclined toward "cleansing" and "purity" is to ask yourself, very honestly and very persistently, "Why do I want to be so pure?" until you get at the deepest possible answer. Usually the reason has to do with a lack of unconditional love from parents and now, internalized, from self.

2. For example, the raw food advocates Herbert Shelton (who died of Parkinson's disease) and T.S. Fry (who died of heart disease).

3. If I seem to be denying personal responsibility and free will, let me hasten to add that the "conditions under which you live" are not themselves arbitrary, but consequent to who you are and what you do. For an in-depth discussion of this apparent paradox, please see the appendix: "The Illness Seeks the Medicine."

4. From the "The Truth That Won't Go Away," an essay about depression in my book, *The Open Secret.*

Chapter 12 - Fasting

1. If the mind-body division seems irreconcilable here, consider what is really meant by a "spiritual practice." The word "practice" should be understood literally. Given the non-dualistic assumption that life itself is a spiritual endeavor, then a spiritual practice is nothing other than a practice for life.

2. There is an important distinction between stimulating the appetite and forcing oneself to eat. Renewed appetite might be a sign that a medicine is working. Thus the benefit of marijuana for cancer and AIDS patients might not be simply that it stimulates the appetite; rather, this potent plant medicine might aid deeper healing, of which improved appetite is an indication.

Chapter 13 - Dieting and Self-Acceptance

1. Paradoxically, "this lifetime" can end before physical death, with "reincarnation in the same body." "Dying before dying" usually entails a rapid transition to a new career, new life partner, new friends, and new location, a transition so acute and so inexorable that it may likened to a birthing. Yet this transition is not a means to accomplish reincarnation in the same body, it is just a byproduct or a sign that it has happened, and one can consciously plan it no more than a fetus can consciously plan his birth.

2. Unless it doesn't. Accepting this possibility is part of letting it be okay.

3. In one sense, something *is* wrong with the body. Obesity and other physical debility may stem from poor nutrition, including prenatal nutrition, rendering the body unable to develop normally. Remember though that even this abnormal development represents the body's very best adaptation to difficult circumstances.

4. Most of us have forgotten how to truly play, so ashamed are we of our natural selves. Sadly, the only time many of us can be uninhibitedly playful is alone with family or lover. When was the last time you rolled on the ground, or ran as fast as you could? Organized competitive sports aren't really the same thing, and even here, participation in sports is in steep decline among post-college adults. As in other realms of modern life, play is increasingly something we pay professionals to do for us.

Chapter 14 - Fat and the Good

1. Examples citing the !Kung are taken from Lee, Richard B. *The Dobe !Kung.* Holt, Rhinehart and Winston, New York, 1984.

2. See for example *The Cholesterol Myths*, by Uffe Ravnskov, MD, PhD.

Chapter 15 - Meat and the Life of the Flesh

1. Some cultures actually attributed the highest, most sacred degree of sentience not to animals or even humans, but to certain plants. Extremely ancient redwoods, banyan trees, and oaks, as well as centuries-old mandrake and ginseng plants, were believed to express a divine intelligence and power. In the cerebral indoor world it is easy to accept the rational arguments why plants could not be sentient, but spend some quiet, attentive time with plants (just being with them, not doing anything) and this rational "knowledge" will give way to a direct "knowing" of plant sentience and the possibility of communication. In an old-growth forest this feeling takes on a palpable presence that even the most insensate materialist can hardly deny. Or maybe I'm just imagining things.

2. Seldom does this happen immediately. Usually the new vegan feels great at first, but after a few months certain aspects of his or her health deteriorate. These symptoms are easily dismissed. Depending on the initial reservoir of health, body type, and motivations, more serious symptoms usually don't set in until after several years. But even when the effects are serious, the vegan might be loath to question her diet because by now her identity and self-esteem are bound up with it; moreover, if she has been proselytizing veganism to others, admitting its failure would be humiliating.

3. Sometimes I am asked, "How dare you speak of 'yoga' and not condemn meat-eating? Doesn't that violate the principle of *ahimsa*, non-violence?" I would respond that I am proposing something much more radically consonant with the spirit of yoga than the mere imposition of an article of dogma. Yoga is, in the words of Patanjali, "the removal of the obstructions of mind," which artificially divide the unitary Self. Rejecting the needs and appetites of the body only strengthens these dividers.

4. Here I am implying a parallel to sexuality. Sometimes spiritual practitioners attempt to reject or deny their sexuality for motives similar to those who reject meat. True, there are yogic and Taoist paths that involve various forms of sexual abstinence, but these are invariably accompanied by techniques to process and transform the sexual energy. When these techniques are carried out, the more physical expressions of sexuality wither away of their own accord. Therefore to refrain from ejaculation or sexual relations in denial of the body's guidance is folly—another form of premature transcendence. The body has a limited capacity for raw sexual energy; anything beyond that capacity must either be transformed or released.

Chapter 16 - Sugar's Sweetness

1. For example when we commit violence, often it seems that "it wasn't really me," that "I was beside myself," that "I was possessed by rage." These locutions express an important truth.

2. To get an idea of the depth of our discomfort, and the degree to which we restrict our connections with others, try the following experiment. Sit or stand a few feet away from another person (agree on this beforehand) and look at each other with an open, unwavering gaze. Do not glaze over or hide behind an expression. Notice the thoughts and feelings that arise. And notice the sensation of centeredness and sweetness when you finish. Many people in our society go years and years without meeting gazes with another human being for more than a couple seconds.

Chapter 17 - The Yoga of Drinking

1. A cup of hot water with lemon or ginger is usually more welcome. When my children get sick though, they often refuse more than half a cup, even of hot liquids. It really depends on the nature of the illness.

2. Human beings ordinarily resist doing vigorous exercise in intense heat. Hot weather makes us feel lethargic. We want to slow down. Intense exercise in extreme heat already conflicts with natural body messages; therefore it is logical that the thirst mechanism is too slow to respond in time to sudden, massive, and rapid fluid loss. That is why the study described says little about ordinary thirst.

3. While compounds such as sulfur, sodium chloride, potassium chloride, or chlorine may be responsible for part of water's taste, there is more to it than that. A significant component of its taste is how the water interacts with the internal environment of the mouth. The taste of water depends on what you've eaten recently, and probably the electrolyte balance of bodily fluids.

4. The sick individual may be innocent of such mistreatment though. I do not mean that if you are sick, it's your fault. Mistreatment can come in the form of environmental pollution, abuse, poverty and other social conditions.

5. There exist rare genetic disorders that might be exceptions to this rule. Apparently there are people who lack the satiety mechanism or have genetically related problems in homeostatic mechanisms governing thirst.

6. Similar reasoning applies to amphetamine-like substances such as Ritalin in the context of school, and to anti-depressant drugs such as Prozac in the context of modern life. When a child has a chronically short attention span in school or is defiant, we tend to blame the child, or the child's brain chemistry. But what if wandering attention is a natural and healthy response to a curriculum not aligned with the child's calling? What if defiance is a natural and healthy response to a school system that crushes creative autonomy? For adults, what if depression—a compulsion to withdraw from life—is a natural and healthy response to the life society presents us with, that is hardly worth living?

Chapter 18 - Supplements

1. This fact was discovered by Dr. Albert Szent-Georgi, who won the Nobel Prize for his discovery of vitamin C, and confirmed in the research of Royal Lee in the 1950s. Why do we equate vitamin C with easily-synthesized ascorbic acid? Could it have anything to do with pharmaceutical company profits?

Chapter 19 - Processing

1. Thoreau, Henry David. *Wild Fruits*. W.W. Norton & Co., New York, 2000. p. 5.

2. If you really want to be strict about it, not even dandelions qualify if you live in America. They are native to the Old World. To the degree that there is not a place on earth with an ecology uncontaminated by exogenous species, it is impossible to find any food that is not somehow affected by human activity.

3. On the other hand, cooking renders the remaining vitamins and minerals more accessible, so that the effect is to increase the food's nutritional value to the modern human. Indeed, many foods such as grains, tubers, and cruciferous vegetables contain harmful substances that are neutralized by cooking.

4. Davidson, Iain; Noble, William (1993) "When did language begin?" In: Burenhult, Goran (ed.) *The First Humans: Human Origins and History to 10,000 B.C.* New York: Harper-Collins Publishers. (p. 46). Cited by Ward Nicholson in "Fire and Cooking in Human Evolution, Rates of Genetic Adaptation to Change, Hunter-Gatherers, and Diseases in the Wild" (http://www.beyondveg.com/nicholson-w/hb/hb-interview2a.shtml#part 2 intro.)

5. *Neanderthals and Modern Humans — A Regional Guide,* by Scott J. Brown, http://www.neanderthal-modern.com/, 2002

6. Some people might object that to really go back to a raw, wild life is impossible because our anatomy and physiology have evolved past that. I would answer that our bodies are far more adaptable than is generally recognized. As I look out on the cows on this wintry day, I am reminded of one example: people who go barefoot in the winter. Yes, you can learn to do this comfortably. I know people who have.

7. It may be that we will someday transcend the technologies of fire, implying that a raw diet could be compatible with a future, more "evolved" state of being which some of us are ready to experience right now. While there has been much misinformation and deception in the area of raw foods diets, I accept that some people do indeed thrive on raw foods without living like a *homo erectus.* Such people are far outnumbered by those debilitated by such a diet, however, and it is very dangerous to dogmatically impose it on yourself.

8. I am thinking here of the classical Chinese distinction between *wen*, the scholar, and *wu*, the warrior. These terms represent cosmic principles that, like other yin-yang polarities, differentiated out of the primordial Tao that might be interpreted here to mean pre-agricultural humanity. *Wen* refers to the civilized side of society—literature, music, and the arts—and is associated with the cultivation of grain.

9. Ethyl-2-methyl butyrate is the main component of the distinctive aroma of an apple (this information comes from Eric Schlosser's article "Why McDonald's Fries Taste So Good," *The Atlantic Monthly*, January, 2000.) However, there are other flavor components as well, which is why attentive tasting can easily distinguish an artificial flavor from the real thing.

10. The reader should be aware that both MSG and artificial flavors may be present in disguised form, the former as hydrolyzed soy protein and autolyzed yeast extract, and the latter as "natural flavors" which are in fact highly

174

purified, chemically refined extracts, albeit from natural sources. For hidden sources of MSG, see *Battling the MSG Myth*, http://www.msgmyth.com.

11. Significantly, three of the biggest growth industries in the 1980s and 1990s were child care, maid services, and ready-to-eat foods. Professional sports—paying people to "play"—is another big growth industry (see note 33).

Appendix I - The Illness Seeks the Medicine

1. In March 2002, Andrea Yates, a Texas woman, was found guilty of capital murder. In June of 2001 she had methodically drowned each of her five children in the bathtub, then called the police and her husband, who was at work.

2. I've come very close to restating the new age cliché, "Everything happens for a purpose," a concept easily open to abuse. The purpose might be beyond human understanding, nor is it necessarily fruitful to try to understand what that purpose may be. Also, see note 4 of Chapter 2.